THE Vegan KITCHEN

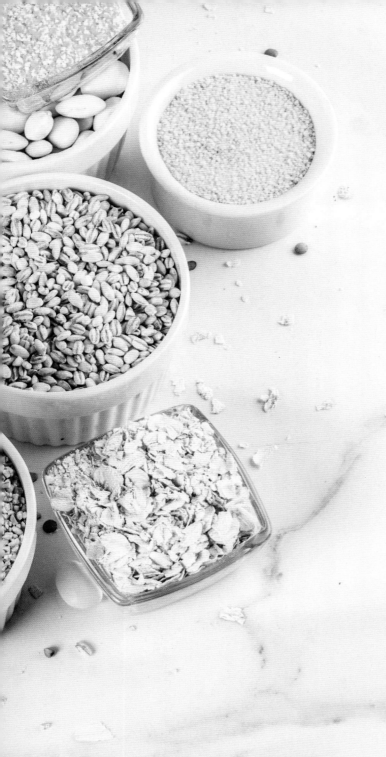

This edition published by OH!
An imprint of the Welbeck Publishing Group
20 Mortimer Street
London W1T 3JW

British Library Cataloguing-in-Publication data
available on request.

ISBN 978-1-85906-458-0

10 9 8 7 6 5 4 3 2 1

Printed in China

THE
Vegan
KITCHEN

OVER *100* ESSENTIAL INGREDIENTS
FOR YOUR PLANT–BASED DIET

Rose Glover and *Laura Nickoll*

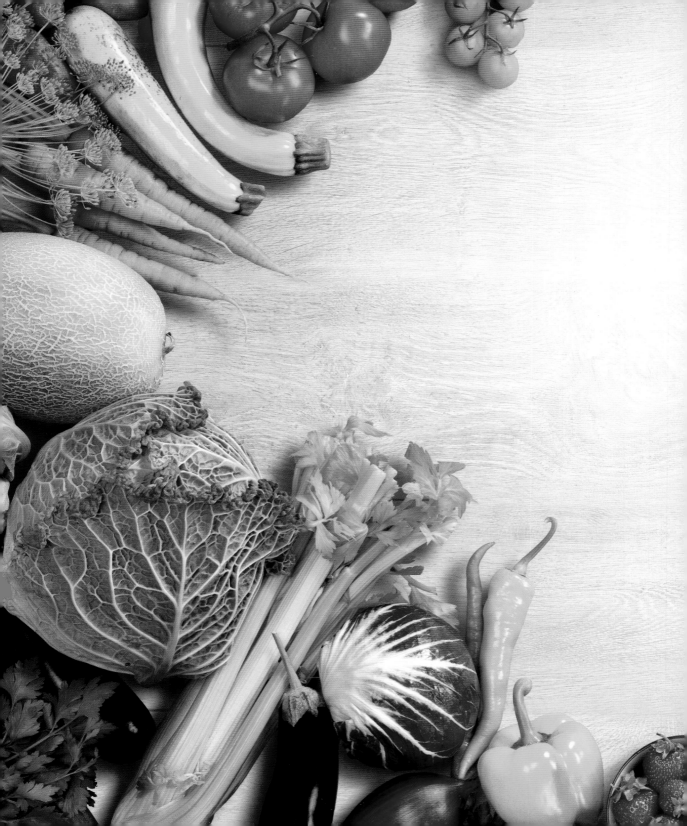

Contents

Introduction

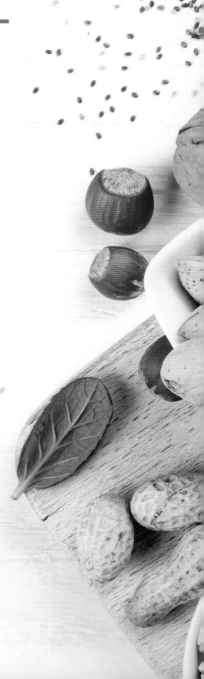

As a lifelong vegetarian, and a vegan for over 20 years, plant-based nutrition and wellness has become my career, my speciality and a personal passion.

After I had graduated from drama school in New York, I packed my suitcase and headed to Los Angeles where I lived and worked as an actress, and it was there that I became truly excited and inspired about health and wellbeing. Although I was living my dream (there's nothing quite like the Californian sun!) I had some niggling health concerns that I was ignoring – I was just hoping they'd go away. And although I enjoyed and relished the Californian lifestyle, I knew in my heart that I wasn't eating quite right as a vegan, and my body was showing me this in all kinds of ways – skin breakouts, unbalanced hormones, a pretty weak immune system and generally feeling lacklustre.

I began to read up on nutrition, and sought out every nutrition book I could get my hands on. Eventually, I started to give my body exactly what it needed to thrive and to feel amazing, all while keeping my diet completely plant-based. I found that a well-planned, healthy vegan diet not only suited my body and helped me feel my best, but it also gave me an immensely rewarding relationship with food while still reflecting my deepest values. Once I was back on home turf in the UK, I was so excited and inspired about specialized nutrition that I decided to throw in the towel on my acting career and go back to university to study nutritional therapy, and I've never looked back.

I believe many people want to adopt a vegan diet, but they simply struggle with how to do it. I hope this book guides, empowers and supports you to venture through unfamiliar territory so that you too can nerd up on plant-based nutrition, feel confident to make informed food choices, enjoy all the flavours and delights of vegan food and become a glowing, happy and healthy example of the vegan lifestyle. Welcome to the journey!

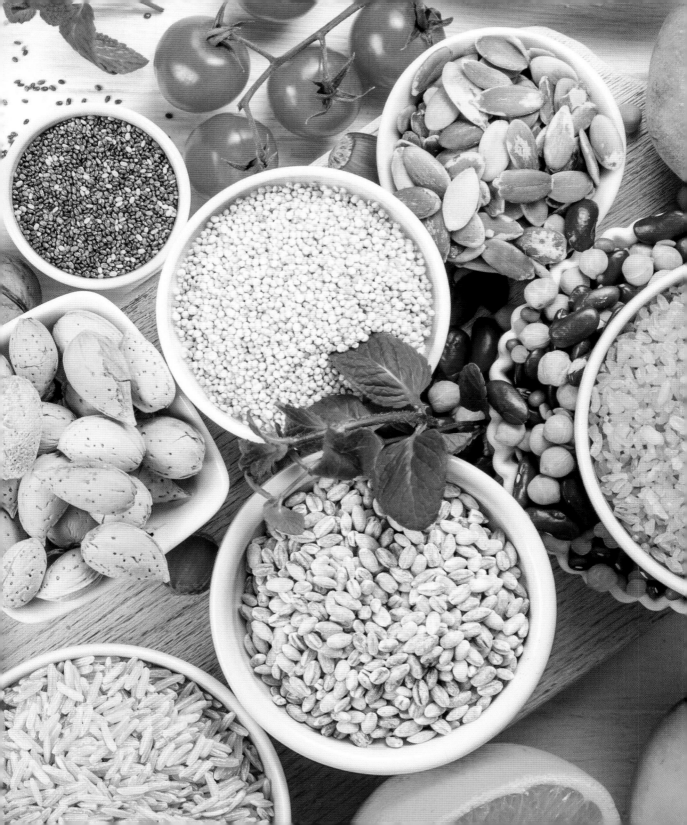

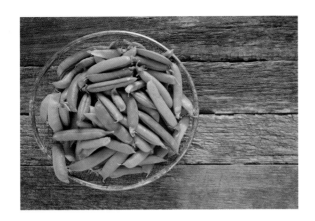

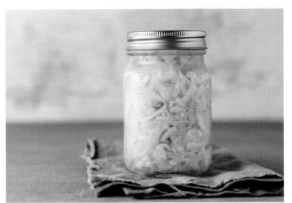

A plant-based

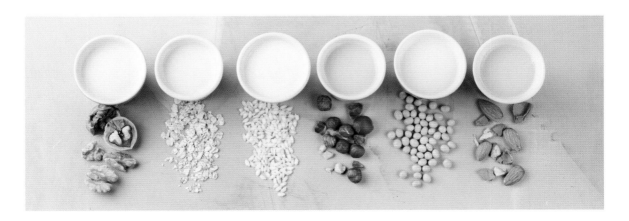

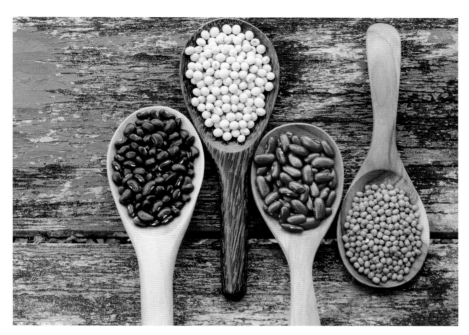

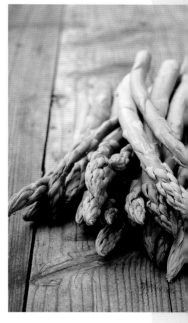

diet

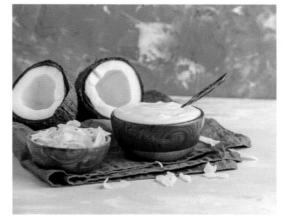

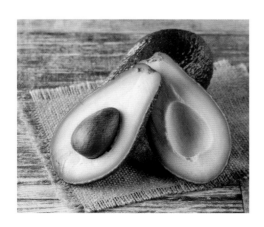

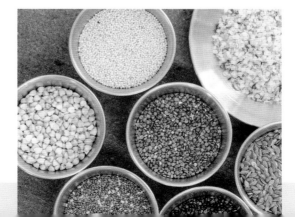

BENEFITS & RISKS OF A PLANT-BASED DIET

What is a vegan diet? Simply put, it's one that excludes meat, fish, eggs, dairy products and animal-derived products such as gelatine and honey, and is based instead entirely on plants, including grains, beans, lentils, vegetables, fruits, nuts, seeds, herbs and spices.

Veganism used to be associated with restrictive and tasteless food, but it is, in fact, a diet which can be healthy, exceedingly satisfying and full of delicious meals and a variety of tastes and textures.

BENEFITS OF A PLANT-BASED DIET

As with any diet, your nutritional requirements depend on your age and state of health, and whether you are pregnant or breastfeeding. Approached in the right way, taking into consideration individual nutritional needs, a vegan diet can be suitable for all stages of the life cycle, including infancy, childhood, adolescence, pregnancy, lactation and older adulthood, and it can be suitable for athletes.

Since a vegan diet is entirely plant-based, it tends to be easier for vegans to load up on the healthy whole grains, legumes (beans and lentils), fruits and vegetables that many people often don't eat enough of. Eating meals based on these food groups can be extremely beneficial. For example, in one study, scientists identified nearly 800 long-lived elderly people from five different communities in Japan, Sweden, Australia and Greece and observed

them for 7 years, tracking their health status and food choices.[1] They found that beans and lentils were the most important dietary predictor of survival among these people, regardless of their ethnicity: for every two-tablespoon increase of daily legume consumption (20g/1oz), there was a staggering 8 per cent reduction in early mortality.

Research also shows that vegan diets, compared to non-vegan diets, tend to be higher in certain nutrients such as fibre, vitamin C, vitamin E, vitamin B_1, magnesium and folate, and are generally lower in calories, cholesterol and saturated fats.[2] Vegans also tend to be slimmer and have lower rates of cardiovascular disease and hypertension. Studies also illustrate that the higher the consumption of animal produce, the higher the risk of Type 2 diabetes and colon cancer.[3] In contrast, research suggests that the higher the intake of colourful fruits and vegetables in one's diet, the lower the risk of certain types of cancers such as breast, prostate, mouth, throat, voice box, oesophagus, stomach and lung.[4]

Even though vegan diets may seem like a new trend, many cultures – both past and present – base their diet on plant foods. It is thought that our prehistoric ancestors started off on a plant-based diet, and eventually went on to consume meat, but only as an occasional feasting food. Fast forward to around 500 BC and the concept of avoiding animal produce was first mentioned by the Greek philosopher Pythagoras, who promoted benevolence to all species, including humans. Around the same time, Siddhārtha Gautama (better known as the Buddha) also advocated vegetarianism, believing that humans should not inflict pain on other animals. To this day, many Buddhists still adhere to a plant-based diet. Indeed, many other religions do the same, including Hindus, Jains,

Seventh Day Adventists and Rastafarians. It was in the West in 1944 that British woodworker Donald Watson rallied together six other non-dairy- and non-egg-eating vegetarians to come up with a word to describe themselves and start a movement, despite much objection. Rejected words included 'dairyban', 'vitan' and 'benevore', but he finally settled on 'vegan', and thus The Vegan Society in the UK was formed.

Nowadays, more and more people are adopting a plant-based diet for a variety of reasons, such as wishing to reduce the cruel and inhumane treatment of animals, or their impact on the environment, or for their own personal health reasons.

RISKS OF A PLANT-BASED DIET

The health benefits of a good vegan diet speak for themselves, but it is possible to be a healthy or unhealthy vegan, just as you can be a healthy or unhealthy meat-eater. Becoming a vegan does not automatically guarantee you good health or a healthy diet. You need more than just avocado on toast and plates of pasta every day, and there is plenty of vegan junk food out there that's marketed as vegan-friendly. It's important to ensure you are making informed decisions and know what nutrients you need to be getting into your diet.

There are a few potential pitfalls when following a vegan diet. In terms of nutrients, vegans tend to have lower levels of vitamin B_{12}, vitamin D, omega-3 fatty acids, calcium and zinc. However, numerous studies have demonstrated that these deficiencies are usually due to poor meal planning. Armed with the knowledge from this book, you can get all the nutrients your body needs to not only survive, but also thrive on a vegan diet.

> The health benefits of
> a good vegan diet speak
> for themselves.

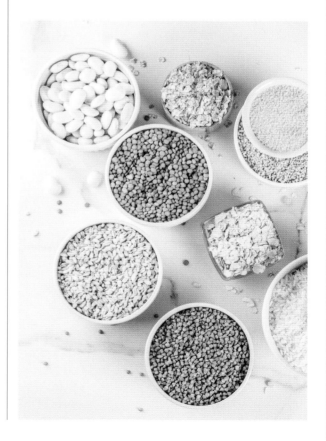

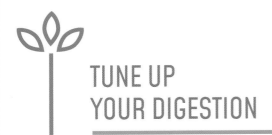

TUNE UP
YOUR DIGESTION

Bloating, indigestion, cramps, constipation... sound familiar? You are not alone. Most people have difficulties with their digestion at some point in their lives. However, an imbalance in the gut can lead to an imbalance elsewhere in the body, so it's important to focus on this vital system. Your wellbeing starts in the gut – you really are what you eat (and absorb).

FOCUS ON FIBRE

Fibre helps 'move things along', so to speak. It has a remarkable ability to swell up and increase in volume by taking on water, which in turn stimulates the stretch receptors in the gut and causes *peristalsis* – wave-like muscle contractions which gently move stools along the intestines to be excreted.

But fibre's other fabulous benefits deserve the spotlight too. As it makes its way through your intestines, it binds to waste products such as excess hormones (especially oestrogen), excess cholesterol and heavy metals such as mercury, and helps you eliminate them. High amounts of hormones or metals in your body increases your risk of developing different types of cancer.

The good news is that plants are high in fibre. The bad news is, if you are a newbie vegan, a sudden increase in fibre intake can cause bloating and stomach discomfort as your body adjusts. If your current diet contains fewer than five portions of fruits and vegetables a day, aim to make the transition relatively gradually and build up your fibre intake (of fruits, vegetables and wholegrains) bit by bit. Your digestion will thank you in the end!

UP YOUR WATER INTAKE

Without adequate quantities of water, fibre can hang around in your gut and get stuck, causing constipation and bloating. Your amazing liver works hard every day to help remove harmful substances and metabolic by-products from your body, dumping them in the gut to be excreted in your stools. If you are constipated, these substances can get reabsorbed back into the body and cause all manner of symptoms, from hormone imbalances to headaches, skin concerns and fatigue.

If you feel thirsty, you may already be dehydrated, so do ensure you drink enough water so that your urine runs clear. Remember, caffeinated drinks don't count, as they act like diuretics, which promote urine excretion and leave you even more dehydrated.

> Without adequate quantities of water, fibre can hang around in your gut and get stuck, causing constipation and bloating.

IT'S ALL ABOUT THE BUGS

Trillions of bacteria colonize your digestive system – they all live together in one big complex ecosystem. Among this clan, there are the so-called 'good' bugs and the 'bad' bugs. Good bugs may include specific strains of bacteria, such as *Lactobacillus acidophilus or Bifidobacterium*, or beneficial yeasts such as *Saccharomyces boulardii*, which can be very beneficial to human health. They can help digest your food and reduce gut inflammation, and they even produce some B vitamins and vitamin K within your gut. So-called bad bugs may include potentially harmful bacteria such as *Escherichia coli* and *Salmonella*, yeasts such as candida, or some parasites, which can cause chronic or acute IBS-type symptoms.

The delicate balance of these bacteria can easily be disrupted, resulting in IBS symptoms such as constipation, diarrhoea and pain in the stomach or digestive system, and has even been linked to arthritis, depression and poor immunity. Imbalances in gut bacteria are very common, and can be caused by any number of things such as sugary foods, food intolerances, stress, medications such as antibiotics, or even a heavy night out on the town.

How to support your gut bacteria balance

- **Probiotics** are live micro-organisms such as beneficial yeasts and bacteria, which can provide many health benefits when consumed, generally by improving or restoring the gut flora. To include these in your diet, stock up on fermented foods such as sauerkraut, non-dairy kefir, miso, vegan-friendly kimchi, kombucha and tempeh. These tangy foods are hosts to a variety of friendly bacteria that your gut will love, and combine well with many savoury dishes.

- Supplement your diet with a good probiotic to help re-inoculate the gut with friendly bacteria. Supplements come in pill, powder or liquid form and are usually available in 1-week, 2-week or 1-month courses. If you are experiencing bloating, gas, diarrhoea or constipation, you may find it useful to take a course and see if your symptoms improve. They can be purchased from most health food stores.

- **Prebiotics** are non-digestible parts of food which act as fuel for the bacteria to munch on so they can multiply and colonize. It's wise to include prebiotics in your diet regularly (ideally three or four times a week). The best food sources include garlic, onions, Jerusalem artichokes, unripe (greenish) bananas and wheat bran.

- Identify food intolerances: if you suspect digestive complaints are caused by a particular food you are eating, try eliminating the suspect food for 30 days. Remember, it can take up to 3 days for a symptom to show up so it may be a good idea to keep a food and symptom diary to help you pinpoint the culprit.

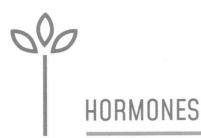

HORMONES

Hormones are chemical messengers that are secreted by various glands in the body, and are responsible for growth, metabolism, sexual and reproductive function, emotions, mood and hunger, and pretty much everything in between. A well-planned vegan diet, supplemented where needed, can provide all the building blocks for hormonal health. Of the many different types, these are the major players.

SEX HORMONES

One major class of hormones are the sex hormones *progesterone*, *testosterone* and *oestrogen*. Sex hormones are derived from cholesterol via a complex chemical process that requires many nutritional co-factors such as vitamin B_5, vitamin C and magnesium.

Progesterone and oestrogen are primarily female hormones, produced by the ovaries and in the adrenal gland. Oestrogen can also be made by fat cells throughout the body. These hormones work in synergy in an intricate and complex system, ideally in perfect harmony. But as many women know, this delicate balance can easily be knocked off kilter, resulting in a range of hormonal conditions and symptoms.

Testosterone is a hormone often associated with males, although smaller amounts are made in the female body

too. Some men suffer from low testosterone levels, mostly caused by issues relating to the glands involved in its production (including the testes, pituitary and hypothalamus glands), which can cause symptoms such as low libido, bone density loss and sleep issues. In contrast, higher testosterone levels in women can cause acne, excess hair on the face and body, and irregular periods.

THYROID HORMONES

The thyroid gland is butterfly shaped and sits low on the front of your neck. It releases two hormones, Triiodothyronine (T_3) and Thyroxine (T_4), which are largely responsible for controlling the metabolism of the body, in turn helping to determine and regulate your weight, energy levels, internal body temperature, skin and hair health. Diseases of the thyroid cause it to make either too much or too little of the hormone, resulting in hyperthyroidism or hypothyroidism. Iodine, selenium and zinc are essential to thyroid health, therefore it's important that vegans get regular sources of these minerals into their diet.

STRESS HORMONES

Three major stress hormones are secreted by the adrenal glands that sit just above the kidneys: adrenaline, norepinephrine and cortisol. Both adrenaline and norepinephrine are responsible for the immediate reactions to stress, and the physical reactions can happen within seconds, such as an increased heart rate and supply of oxygen to the muscles, sharpened mental focus and a surge of energy. These processes are cleverly designed by the body so that it can respond when it feels there is an imminent threat to its safety. Cortisol, on the other hand, is the stress hormone released in response to chronic stress, such as the everyday pressures of modern life. In optimal amounts, cortisol helps maintain fluid balance, blood pressure, immunity and growth. However, problems arise when too much cortisol is released over a longer period of time, resulting in a suppressed immune system, increased blood pressure and blood sugars, acne, obesity and more.

B vitamins, vitamin C, magnesium and healthy fats are all essential for helping your body regulate your stress response and support your adrenal glands. Fruits and vegetables are nutritional powerhouses that contain many of the elements your body needs to support your hormones.

HOW TO SUSTAIN HORMONAL BALANCE

Even the smallest imbalance in hormones can have a major impact on your body. While some people can cope with these changes relatively smoothly, others feel they are dragging their bodies through it all, kicking and screaming. Hormones can dictate your weight, skin health, mental health and vitality. Luckily, you can use the healing power of foods to help overcome the turmoil of this complex system.

OPTIMIZE GUT FUNCTION
Gut health is paramount. The gut is where all your used and excess hormones are bound to fibrous material for elimination from the body. If you suffer from poor gut function, be it chronic constipation, indigestion or diarrhoea, the hormonal balance within the body can easily become imbalanced. Gut health is very individual to the person, therefore it's important to pinpoint and solve what triggers any gut issues (see page 13).

Adaptogenic herbs and spices

Specific adaptogenic herbs, spices and even some fungi can work with your body to help it adapt and recalibrate during times of physical or emotional stress by modulating the release of stress hormones from the adrenal glands – helping to support your body through any changes to your circumstances or surroundings. These include ashwaganda, astragalus, ginseng, liquorice root, holy basil, some mushrooms and rhodiola. These can be taken in supplement form, in teas or added to meals. For example, ashwagandha is great for people who find it hard to unwind, and can be both calming and energizing. Whereas evidence suggests rhodiola encourages strong mental and cognitive function.

MANAGE INFLAMMATION
Inflammation can be the cause of many hormonal imbalances. Aim to have a small daily serving of nuts and seeds, especially walnuts, chia and flaxseeds, to ensure you are consuming essential fats. These fats are crucial for the health of hormone receptor sites on cell membranes and for the production of anti-inflammatory compounds within the body.

Fact:

The 'bioavailability' of a nutrient is defined as how well the body absorbs nutrients into the bloodstream from the gastrointestinal tract so you can utilize them in your cells all around your body. Just because a food is high in some nutrients doesn't necessarily mean your body is capable of absorbing all of them!

BALANCE BLOOD SUGAR LEVELS

Sugar and refined carbohydrates are not your friend. They can contribute to blood sugar imbalances, which throw the other hormones in your body, such as cortisol and sex hormones, offkilter. Excess sugar is also converted to fat, and as fat cells make oestrogen, this can also contribute to hormone imbalances.

SUPPORT THE LIVER

If your liver isn't functioning at its best, it may mean that hormone clearance from the body is inhibited. Your liver makes 80 per cent of the cholesterol in your body; many major hormones are made from cholesterol, such as all the sex hormones and the stress hormone cortisol. To support your liver, eat plenty of cruciferous vegetables such as broccoli, cauliflower, kale, cabbage and Brussel sprouts, as these contain a compound called *glucosinolates*, which support the removal of excess oestrogen and other used hormones from the body. It's also a good idea to steer away from consuming too much alcohol, fried foods and sugar as they can be a heavy burden on your liver.

REDUCE XENOESTROGENS (HORMONE DISRUPTORS)

Xenoestrogens are chemicals found in plastics that we used to bottle our drinks and wrap our food, as well as everyday cosmetics and cleaning products, so try to use natural products if you can, and avoid plastic packaging. Use unbleached tea bags, toilet paper and tampons.

ADJUST YOUR LIFESTYLE

Even small changes to your lifestyle can have a big impact in the long run. Have some stress management techniques up your sleeve, such as meditation, mindfulness and journalling, and try to incorporate regular, moderate amounts of exercise into your week. Even if you just walk a little more than usual, the key is to get moving!

What is inflammation?

It's a bit of a buzzword nowadays, but what exactly is it and why does it affect us so much? Inflammation is an immune response which is initiated in the body to help us fight off anything that may do us harm, such as injuries, infections, viruses, food intolerances or stress. Ideally, this immune process is triggered and the body releases inflammatory cells that then repair or rebalance the issue, the inflammation dies down and the job is done. This type of inflammation is a good thing – it's there to protect and heal us, and we need it.

However, often this inflammatory response doesn't die down, and inflammation simmers in the background and manifests in all sorts of different ways in the body. This low-grade chronic 'background' inflammation may be due to the fact that many of us are living quite inflammatory lifestyles compared to even our most recent ancestors. So much has changed in the way we live, even in the last 100 years. Not eating enough anti-inflammatory foods (think colourful veggies and omega-3 fats), the industrialization of food (highly processed and non-organic foods), soil depletion, medications, pollution and the mammoth amount of stress that modern life entails, may all contribute to inflammation. This can manifest in all sorts of ways in the body and contribute to imbalances such as hormonal issues, acne, rheumatoid arthritis, autoimmune conditions, depression and anxiety.

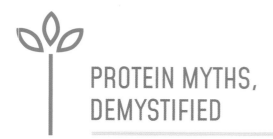

PROTEIN MYTHS, DEMYSTIFIED

Protein is considered somewhat of a superhero macronutrient because of its crucial role in almost every mechanism in the body.

The multitude of functions include creating the structure, growth and repair mechanisms of your bones, blood, skin, organs, hormones, muscles and just about everything else in between.

Protein is made up of building blocks called amino acids. There are twenty different amino acids, nine of which are called essential amino acids – these must be obtained from food (your body is very clever, and can actually create the non-essential amino acids itself when it needs to). A food that contains all nine essential amino acids is often referred to as a 'complete' protein. Meat, dairy and eggs all fall into this category. Some plant foods, such as quinoa, soya foods, buckwheat and hemp are also complete proteins. Other plant foods such as legumes, vegetables and grains also contain essential amino acids, but are low in – or lack – one or more amino acid, making them 'incomplete' proteins.

It used to be thought that vegetarians needed to combine specific foods at each meal to get sufficient protein – a rather arduous task. This is simply not true. By eating a good variety of legumes, grains and vegetables daily, you'll be getting enough protein. Your body can pool together different amino acids from various sources and re-create the protein it needs, as necessary: it simply re-strings the amino acids into the protein it is making.

Almost all plant foods contain proteins in various degrees, but beans, lentils, nuts and seeds are particularly good sources. Some vegetables that are especially rich sources of amino acids include broccoli, peas, spinach, asparagus, artichokes, potatoes, sweet potatoes and Brussels sprouts. Protein deficiency is often seen in underdeveloped nations, but is very rare in western cultures. To become deficient in protein, you would need to either live off a diet that consisted solely of refined and processed foods, or eat a diet that didn't meet your calorie needs.

TOO MUCH OF A GOOD THING CAN BE A BAD THING

Protein is a bit of a buzzword lately, especially when it comes to marketing and selling food and drink products. Many lifestyle magazines also continue to wrongly assert that protein bars, shakes and lots of animal protein are needed for good health and a six-pack.

tip

Consuming a good-quality, low-processed protein powder is perfectly fine every now and then, just don't rely on it for your protein needs. Your body can only absorb 20–25g (1oz) of protein at a time, so stick to the recommended serving size.

In fact, chronically over-consuming protein can be detrimental to your health. The kidneys work very hard to break down the nitrogenous waste from excessive protein intake, which over time can lead to kidney stones and renal diseases. Countless studies also suggest that overconsumption of protein is associated with higher rates of cancer, osteoporosis, liver function disorders and coronary heart disease.

Many people transitioning to a vegan diet rely too heavily on mock meats to get their protein fix. These foods can be highly processed, and high in salt and refined ingredients. If you are tempted to do the same, consider this first: what exactly is it you are craving? Texture? Saltiness? Fat? Experiment with vegan recipes using whole foods to satisfy your cravings. For example, miso, kombu (Japanese seaweed) and dried mushrooms are just some plant-based foods that provide the taste of umami – a strong savoury flavour often found in meat and dairy products.

STRAIGHT TALK ABOUT SOYA

When it comes to health, soya foods are both vilified and celebrated. Even in large media publications, debate, controversy and confusion remains as to whether this

How much protein do you need?

To figure out your protein needs, use this simple formula. If you are an adult, multiply your weight in kilograms by 0.8 to get your required grams of protein per day, or 0.36 grams per pound. For example, a woman weighing 60kg (132lb) would need 48 grams of protein daily (60 x 0.8 = 48, 132 x 0.36).

PROTEIN INTAKE GUIDELINES:

Infants:	1.5g/kg/day
Ages 1–3:	1.1g/kg/day
Ages 4–13:	0.95g/kg/day
Ages 14–18:	0.85g/kg/day
Adults 19 and above:	0.8g/kg/day
Pregnancy (pre-pregnancy weight):	1.1g/kg/day
Lactating:	1.1g/kg/day

It is good to calculate your needs, but after you've done it, put the calculator down! You don't need to weigh and count your protein intake every single day to make sure you are reaching your protein needs. Focus instead on following a wholefood diet with plenty of variety.

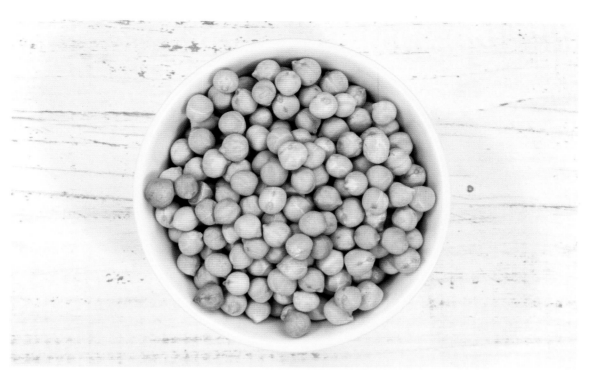

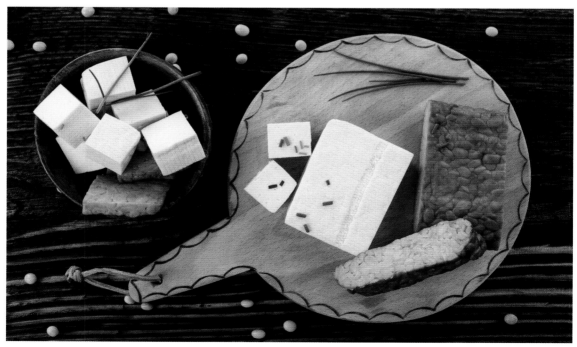

humble little bean is friend or foe. Is it safe to consume it if you have a family history of breast cancer? Or, conversely, does it actually reduce your risk of getting cancer?

Here's the lowdown: Soya foods can be an important part of a vegan diet, as they contain all nine essential amino acids, as well as B vitamins, fibre, potassium and magnesium. Soya beans also contain a class of phytoestrogens called *isoflavones*, a compound which molecularly looks very similar to the female hormone *oestrogen*, but has much weaker effects on the body. High levels of oestrogen have been linked to an increased risk of breast cancer. However, soya foods don't contain high enough levels of phytoestrogens to increase breast cancer risk. In fact, a range of studies now show that whole soya foods such as tofu, tempeh, miso and edamame beans don't increase cancer risk at all, and may actually lower the risk of both prostate and breast cancer. Therefore, you can enjoy a moderate amount of unprocessed or lightly processed soya without concern. A moderate amount is one or two servings a day, for example a serving could be a cup of soya milk or roughly 100g of tofu. As with any diet, don't rely too heavily on one food for the majority of your calories: aim to have soya foods two or three times a week and ensure you are getting a variety of other foods in your diet.

Concentrated forms of phytoestrogens, such as soya or isoflavone supplements, however, may be a cause for concern so give these a miss if you have had breast cancer or have a family history of it. This is because these supplements can be extremely concentrated forms of processed soya, the effects of which are not entirely clear

Fact:

Kidney beans and soya beans can't be sprouted as they are toxic when they are raw (see pages 92 and 98). Once cooked, however, these beans make a great protein-rich addition to any dish.

for your long-term health. However, the general consensus is that breast cancer survivors or those with breast cancer in the family may safely eat whole soya foods such as edamame, tofu or soya milk/yoghurt, or fermented soya foods such as miso or tempeh, in moderation.

Also, try to avoid soya protein isolates – a highly processed offspring to soya that shows up as an added ingredient in many foods. Soya protein isolate is chemically engineered, a process that strips all other nutrients from the soya bean except protein, making this by-product highly processed. If in doubt, always read the label and aim to eat foods – all foods – in their whole state as often as you can. The health benefits of any legume or vegetable stem from the plant's various components being eaten at the same time. Therefore, aim to avoid highly processed soya products, soya supplements or soya additives.

DIGESTING LEGUMES

Beans can cause excess gas and a variety of other digestive complaints in some people, which can be off-putting. Here are some strategies you can use to radically improve digestion and increase the bioavailability of nutrients from beans and lentils.

SOAK THEM: Soak dried beans in double the volume of water overnight, or for 24 hours. Change the soaking water once in that time. Drain, rinse and use fresh water to cook.

SPROUT THEM: You could leave them a little longer to soak for a few days until they start to sprout (or until a little

tip

Over 90 per cent of soya crops are genetically modified. Buying organic ensures you are getting non-GM soya.

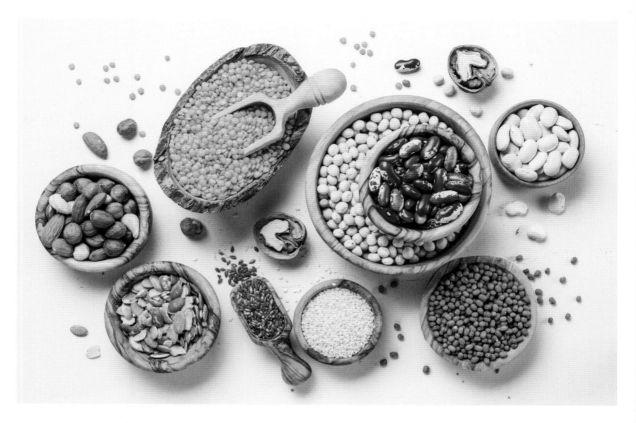

tail appears on the bean) - remember to still change the soaking water often in that time.

COOK THEM LONG AND SLOW: After soaking, cook them slowly. A slow cooker works well for this. Cooking beans all day allows plenty of time for the heat to break down those hard-to-digest fibres.

START SLOWLY: Gradually increase your consumption over the course of a few weeks. Start with 1 tablespoon every few days and slowly build up to half a cup every couple days.

FLAVOUR THEM: Use spices such as fennel, turmeric, ginger, cumin and turmeric when cooking your beans. These spices can help improve digestion, and they add tons of flavour to the beans.

USING TINNED PRE-COOKED BEANS: These may cause a little more gas than cooking your own beans, but rinsing them under cold water in a colander for 1 minute helps remove substances that can cause gas and discomfort.

Still struggling? Try taking a digestive enzyme supplement which contains *alpha-galactosidase* – an enzyme that helps break down the carbohydrates in beans into simpler sugars to make them easier to digest.

Soak dry beans with a strip of kombu, which contains the enzyme needed to break down the carbohydrate molecules that can cause digestive issues.

TYPICAL PROTEIN CONTENT OF VEGAN FOODS

*Note: This is based on a 100-gram serving of each food, which is not necessarily the average serving you might have. For example, a typical tin of drained chickpeas is 240g (8oz) and a typical baked potato weighs 150–200g (5–7oz).

FOOD	AVERAGE PROTEIN / 100g
ALMONDS	21g (0.74oz)
TEMPEH	20g (0.7oz)
CASHEWS	18g (0.63oz)
BUTTER BEANS, COOKED	9g (0.32oz)
PLAIN OATCAKES	9g (0.32oz)
TOFU	8g (0.28oz)
GREEN, BROWN AND RED LENTILS	8g (0.28oz)
CHICKPEAS, COOKED	8g (0.28oz)
GREEN PEAS, COOKED	5.5g (0.19oz)
BROCCOLI, COOKED	3.3g (0.12oz)
BROWN BASMATI RICE, COOKED	3.3g (0.12oz)
ASPARAGUS, STEAMED	3g (0.1oz)
POTATO, BAKED	2.5g (0.09oz)

Source: Composition of foods integrated dataset (CoFID). Public Health England.

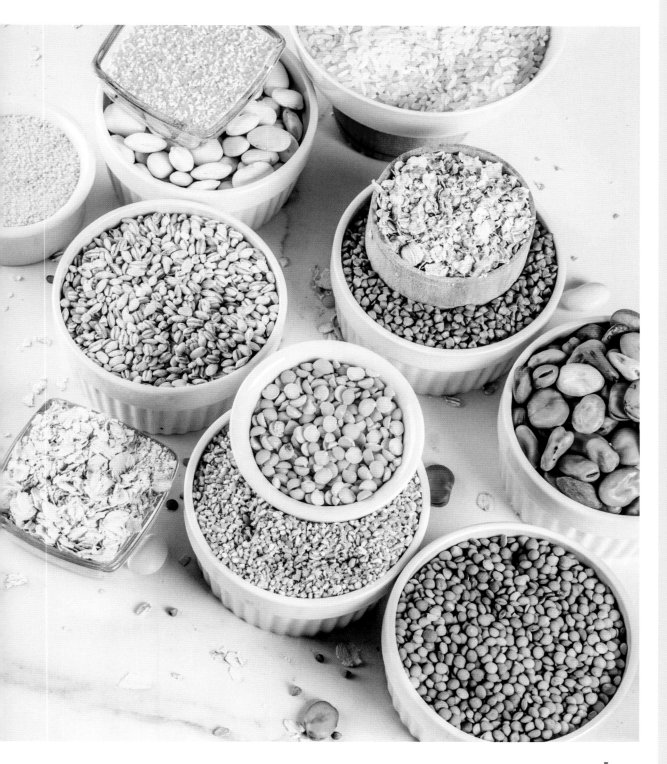

FATS

Some fats are potentially harmful to health, while others are essential for good health. There are four main types of fats we can get from food; trans fats, saturated, monounsaturated and polyunsaturated fats.

TRANS FATS

Let's start with the baddies. Trans fats are chemically altered fats from vegetable oils that are modified by a process called hydrogenation to make food solid at room temperature (such as margarines), extend a product's shelf life and increase the melting point of fat (for deep-frying). They also occur naturally in small amounts in meat and dairy products. From a health perspective, they are a disaster and can significantly increase the risk of heart attacks, strokes and Type 2 diabetes. In 2013, the US Food and Drug Administration (FDA) stated that they are no longer generally recognized as safe for human consumption. However, they can still be found in food. Sources include processed and deep-fried foods, cookies, doughnuts, muffins, pies, shortening and some margarines. Quite simply, if you see the words 'hydrogenated' or 'partially hydrogenated' on a packet of food, avoid it.

SATURATED FATS

These fats are mostly found in animal foods like fatty meats and dairy products such as butter, lard and cheese. They can raise the level of cholesterol in your blood and they've been linked to the increase of heart disease, stroke and some cancers. General medical advice is to limit these types of fats in the diet. The only plant sources of saturated fat are coconut oil, palm kernel oil and palm oil. It's fine to cook with coconut oil every now and then – as with everything, moderation is key.

MONOUNSATURATED FATS

These are generally considered good fats and they can be very beneficial to your health. Sound scientific evidence suggests they can reduce blood pressure and enhance blood flow.[5] Studies also show that when polyunsaturated and monounsaturated fats replace saturated fats in the diet, heart disease risk significantly drops.[6] Sources include most nuts and seeds, olives and olive oil, sesame oil, peanut oil, canola oil and avocados.

tip

Not all oils are good for cooking with. Use cold-pressed oils, virgin oils and walnut and flax oils to drizzle over vegetables once cooked, or use them in a salad dressing.

POLY-UNSATURATED FATS: TIME FOR AN OIL CHANGE

Two essential fats fall into this category: alpha-linolenic acid and linoleic acid (also known as omega-3 and omega-6). Your body can't produce these fats on its own, therefore you must get them from food.

Omega-3s form an integral part of all cell membranes and provide a starting point for the processes which make hormones, and regulate blood, heart and genetic function. Essentially, omega-3s do for your body what oil does for a car – it keeps it running smoothly. Sound science suggests that these fats can help in the management of a number of diseases such as rheumatoid arthritis, Crohn's disease, ulcerative colitis, psoriasis, lupus, cardiovascular diseases, MS, migraines and hormonal imbalances. These essential fats also have a significant impact on brain health, with studies showing they have an ability to reduce anxiety, depression and stress, and improve mood, memory and concentration.

Omega-3 fats come in three different forms: Eicosapentenoic acid (EPA), docosahexenoic acid (DHA), which come from oily fish, and the plant-based alpha-linolenic acid (ALA). When you eat ALA, your body converts it into EPA and DHA, which then get converted into anti-inflammatory compounds that your body can utilize. Here lies a potential issue: it is estimated that just 5–10 per cent of ALA is converted to EPA and just 2–5 per cent to DHA. In fact, studies show that vegans and vegetarians tend to have lower blood levels of EPA and DHA than fish-eaters. Therefore, to ensure adequate levels, it's vital for vegans to ensure they are consuming plant-based omega-3 every day. Sources include walnuts, ground flaxseeds, chia seeds, seaweeds, green leafy vegetables, walnut oil and flax oil. A vegan DHA/EPA supplement may also be useful.

Omega-6 fats are also important for the health of our brains and structure of our cells. However, while omega-3 is highly anti-inflammatory in the body, excess amounts of omega-6 can lead to the production of pro-inflammatory hormones. Please note, while it's very difficult to get too much omega-3 through diet alone, omega-3 supplementation may decrease the blood's ability to clot, so speak to your doctor if you have any concerns.

Anthropological and epidemiological studies indicate that humans evolved on a diet with a ratio of 1:1 omega-6 to omega-3. In contrast, in our modern western culture, it is estimated that the ratio is more like 16:1, which is thought to promote the development of many inflammatory and autoimmune diseases. Omega-6 fats are found in vegetable oils, sunflower oil, soya bean oil, sesame oil and corn oil – oils that are often used in the manufacture of processed foods. Some nuts, seeds, meat, dairy and eggs also contain omega 6 fats. That doesn't mean you should stop eating nuts – you just need to ensure you consume plenty of omega-3 in your diet while limiting the intake of omega-6-rich oils found mostly in packaged foods.

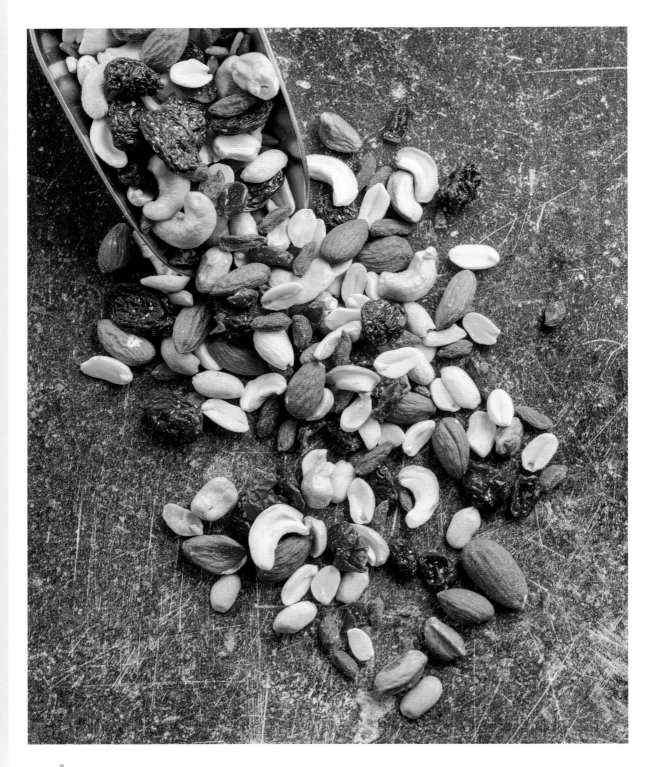

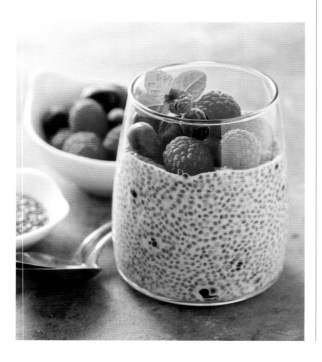

WAYS YOU CAN INCREASE YOUR PLANT-BASED OMEGA-3 INTAKE

1. Breakfast is a great time to eat those omega-rich seeds. Add a tablespoon of ground or soaked flaxseeds to your porridge, granola, plant yoghurt or smoothie in the morning.
2. Go nuts! Sprinkle walnuts and pecans liberally on salads for extra texture. Dry-toast them gently in a pan first, to bring out their flavour and give them crunch.
3. Make your own omega-3 trail mix. Combine walnuts, pecans, pumpkin seeds, almonds and dried cranberries (add dark chocolate chips as a treat).
4. Make a yummy anti-inflammatory nut butter. Blitz walnuts in a high-speed blender with a splash of walnut oil, along with a sprinkle of salt and ground cinnamon, until smooth. Spread on toast or apple wedges for a perfect snack.
5. Use walnut oil or flax oil in salad dressings for an extra anti-inflammatory hit.
6. Make chia seed pudding – it works for breakfast, dessert or a sweet snack. Simply mix chia seeds with oats in plant-based milk or yoghurt, add fresh fruit such as grated apple, berries or chopped mango, and leave to soak in the fridge overnight. In the morning, add extra fruit, a drizzle of maple syrup and some crunchy seeds or almonds. Make your chia seed pudding in a Tupperware for breakfast on the go.
7. Use seaweed flakes in cooked or cold dishes, or sprinkle on top of food instead of salt for an omega-3 boost.
8. Try a plant-based omega-3 supplement specified as EPA/DHA, which is the most bioavailable form.

CARBOHYDRATES

Are carbs healthy? Or are they fattening? When it comes to this macronutrient, there is a lot of carb-confusion and carb-phobia. The fact is, not all carbs are created equal. It's the type, quality and quantity of carbohydrates in the diet that counts.

Unfortunately, foods made with processed and refined carbohydrate, such as doughnuts, cakes and cookies, all get lumped together in the same category as unprocessed carbs such as wholegrains and starchy foods (e.g. brown rice, beans, potatoes and other root vegetables).

Let's break it down. There are two main types of carbohydrates in food: simple and complex.

Fact:

Time to ditch the sugar. Sugar is highly addictive, both physically and emotionally. Studies show it may be just as addictive as cocaine.[7] Sugar contributes to weight gain (many low-fat products are unfortunately loaded with sugar) and may increase the risk of heart disease, cancer and diabetes, premature ageing and Alzheimer's.

and minerals and form an essential part of the diet. Aim to get your simple sugars from these sources.

Remember: Processed and convenience foods that no longer resemble their original state can lack a healthy nutritional profile and should be left off the shopping list!

SIMPLE CARBOHYDRATES

These are carbohydrates that have been refined and stripped of many of their nutrients such as fibre, B vitamins and minerals. Examples include white rice, white bread and white pasta, as well as products made from refined flours such as baked goods. White sugar is also a simple carb that is often added to fizzy drinks, yoghurts, cakes, cookies and breakfast cereals, among many other products. The sugars in maple syrup, agave and coconut nectar are all simple sugars, too. This is the type of carbohydrate that should be reduced in the diet for optimal health. Natural simple sugars found in fruit and vegetables don't count because they come all packaged up with fibre, vitamins

COMPLEX CARBOHYDRATES

Also known as starches, foods such as wholegrain cereals, brown bread, brown rice and wholegrain pasta all fall into this category. When these foods are in their wholefood state (as opposed to their white, refined versions), they qualify as a complex carb and can provide a slow and steady release of energy throughout the day. Starchy foods are a good source of energy: they also provide fibre, calcium, iron and B vitamins and are essential for a balanced diet. These foods also tend to be rich in fibre, which keeps you feeling full so you're less likely to overeat. On average, most people don't consume enough fibre, so increasing these foods could be very beneficial.

BALANCING BLOOD SUGAR LEVELS

In essence, the difference between simple and complex carbs is how quickly they are digested and absorbed. Simple carbs are absorbed faster, releasing their sugars relatively quickly into the bloodstream, which can set you off on an energy and cravings rollercoaster that can last all day long. This is also known as a blood sugar imbalance, which can impact your mood, weight, sleep, energy levels and concentration and much more.

We've all experienced a blood sugar low – that familiar mid-afternoon slump when your energy and concentration plummet and cravings kick in. If this sounds familiar to you, bin those sugary cereals, white breads/pastas and sugary teas and instead opt for complex carbohydrates, which are much more slowly absorbed. Good snack options to help balance blood sugar levels include: nuts and seeds; low-sugar fruit such as apples, pears and berries; nut butters spread on wholegrain crackers or on fruit slices; rye bread or raw veggie sticks with hummus; roasted chickpeas; or edamame beans.

tip

Include a good source of protein in every meal and snack. Protein helps release the carbohydrates even more slowly into your bloodstream, keeping you feeling fuller and contented for longer.

Blood sugar 101

What actually happens inside the body during a blood sugar high or low?

Carbohydrates are broken down in the body into a sugar called glucose, which is carried around in the bloodstream and transported to cells, where it is either used as energy or stored as fat. Your blood only likes a certain amount of glucose in it at any one time – about 1–2 teaspoons. If you consume more than this, your pancreas produces the hormone insulin, which then goes about removing this sugar from the bloodstream.

If your blood sugar level rises too rapidly, as is often the case when you eat a load of refined carbs or sugar, your body can end up releasing too much insulin in a bid to try and get your levels back to 'normal' again. This can then cause your blood sugars to drop, causing a blood sugar low. If you consume sugar on a regular basis, your cells can become a little lazy and stop reacting to the presence of insulin which can lead to diseases such as Type 2 diabetes.

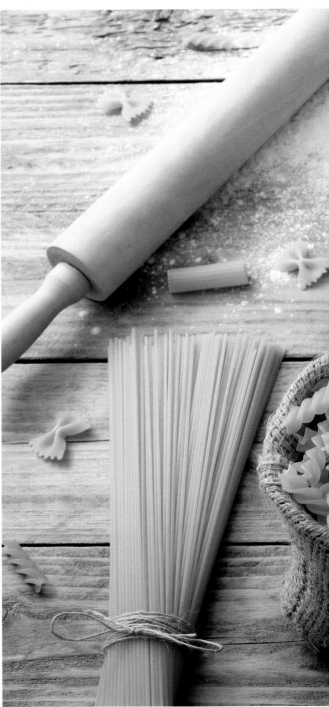

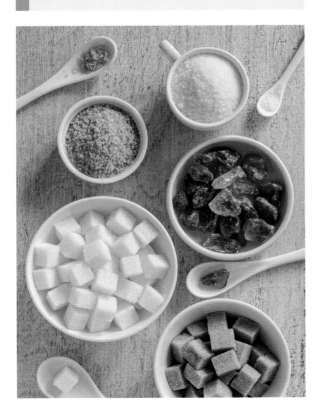

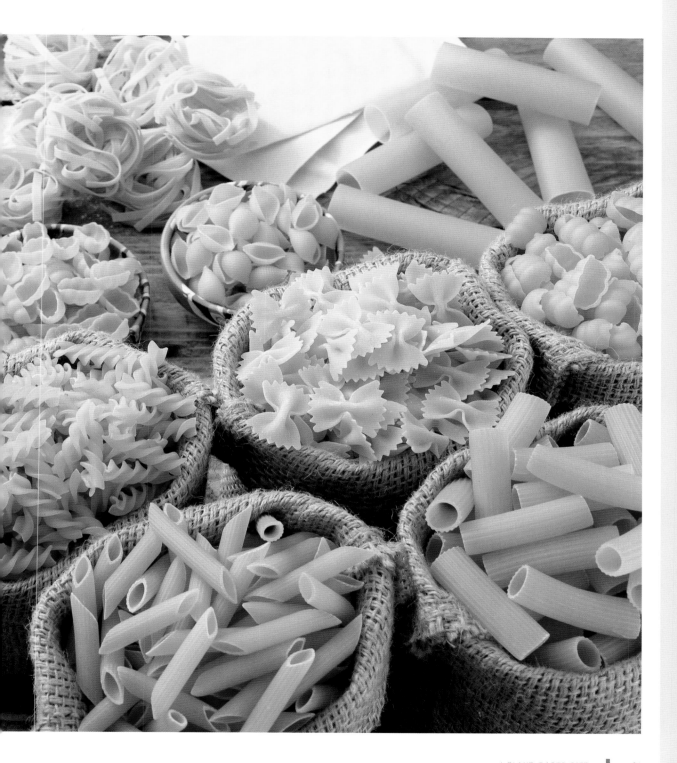

MINERALS

Minerals are inorganic substances that are required by the body to perform a variety of functions to keep us alive.

Some minerals, called *macro*-minerals, are required in larger quantities than others (e.g. calcium, magnesium and phosphorus). Others, the *trace* minerals, are required in smaller amounts but are still essential to health (e.g. iron, zinc and selenium).

Let's focus on four minerals that vegans need to pay special attention to: iron, zinc, calcium and iodine.

IRON

It is commonly thought that vegetarians and vegans are more at risk of iron deficiency than meat-eaters, however studies actually show that vegans and vegetarians who eat a varied and well-balanced diet are at no greater risk. Iron deficiency is the number one deficiency worldwide and can affect anyone, vegan and meat-eater alike.

There are two types of iron you can get from food – *haem* iron from meat and *non-haem* iron from plants. So why does plant-based iron get a bad rap? Vegan foods contain non-haem iron in abundance, however it can be a little trickier for your body to absorb it, in contrast to haem iron. Sources include green leafy vegetables, beans, lentils, tofu and seeds such as chia, flax, hemp and pumpkin seeds.

How to improve absorption of non-haem iron

- Avoid drinking coffee and tea (including black and green tea) within an hour of eating your meals. They contain tannic acid, a compound which can inhibit iron absorption.

- Eat vitamin C-rich foods in the same meal as iron-rich foods. The vitamin C can increase the absorption of the iron by up to four times. Sources of vitamin C include sweet (bell) peppers, citrus fruits, tomatoes, potatoes and green leafy vegetables.

- Cooking your food in a cast-iron pan can increase the food's iron content. Foods cooked must be both water-based and acidic (such as tomatoes or sweet and sour sauce) in order to absorb the iron from the pan. This form of iron can be used by our cells pretty much the same way as iron from food is. Strange but true!

ZOOM IN ON ZINC

Some studies suggest that vegans' zinc intake may be a little on the low side, but this is found mostly in vegans who don't meet their daily calorie needs. Therefore, it's vital you are consuming enough nutrient-dense calories per day to meet your mineral needs. Your calorie needs vary depending on your age and physical activity, but as a guide an average adult man needs 2,500kcal daily, while an average woman needs 2,000kcal. However, unless you feel you may be under-consuming or over-consuming your calorie intake, there's no need to count how many calories you are consuming daily.

Plant foods do contain plenty of zinc, but they also contain an anti-nutrient called *phytic acid*, which may inhibit the body's ability to effectively absorb zinc, as well as other minerals like iron.

CALCIUM

There's more to calcium status in the body than how much calcium you actually *consume*. It concerns how much you *absorb*, and how much you *lose*, and all three factors affect bone density. For example, high protein diets that are especially high in sulphur-containing amino acids can negatively affect calcium balance by increasing calcium loss from the bones. Meat is considered to have a strong negative effect on calcium balance because it is a concentrated form of protein, and has particularly high levels of sulphur-containing amino acids. Vegan diets which are high in protein powders, especially soya protein, can also contribute to calcium loss. Of course, protein is an essential nutrient, but consuming excessive amounts can have drawbacks in terms of bone health (see also pages 17–18).

IODINE

Worldwide iodine deficiency is a global public health concern, affecting nearly one out of every three people worldwide. Research shows that there may be an increased risk for individuals with plant-based diets to be deficient, especially those following the raw food diet. Iodine can be a difficult nutrient to find in a vegan diet, as iodine content varies widely depending on the soil in which the plants are grown. Good amounts of iodine are consistently found in only very few foods, such as dairy (iodine solutions are used to clean the cows' teats and dairy equipment, so it ends up in the milk) and seafood (including seaweed).

How to reduce phytates in your food

- Soak beans, grains and seeds for a few hours before cooking them. Soaking also makes them easier to digest and reduces the chance of gas and bloating.

- Sprout beans, grains and seeds and add them to salads or snacks (see page 95). Sprouting dramatically increases the nutritional content of foods. For example, the vitamin C content in germinated lentils increases by 17.5 times and by 8.5 times in mung beans. It is also a great way to increase absorption of both iron and zinc.

- Incorporating fermented foods such as miso and tempeh into your diet significantly reduces phytates in soya foods. Fermented foods are also rich in enzymes and probiotics, which help you break down and digest other foods eaten at the same meal

- Choose leavened grain products, i.e. bread, over unleavened foods, i.e. crackers, as leavened foods help break down phytate in these grain products.

tip

Aim to limit your intake of salty foods – use herbs, spices or seaweed flakes to enhance flavour instead. High amounts of sodium can increase calcium loss. For every gram of sodium the kidneys excrete, 23–26g (0.8–0.9oz) of calcium is lost.

Essential minerals and where to find them

MINERAL	FUNCTIONS
CALCIUM	Essential for healthy bones and teeth. Helps transmit messages from the brain to the nervous system.
PHOSPHORUS	Together with calcium it is essential for healthy bone and tooth structure.
MAGNESIUM	Essential mineral present in all human tissues. Needed for the activation of many enzymes and essential in nerve and muscle function.
SODIUM	Responsible for regulating the body's water content and electrolyte balance.
POTASSIUM	Vital for regulating the body's water content and electrolyte balance and the normal functioning of cells, including nerves.
IRON	Essential for the formation of hemoglobin in red blood cells. Vital in many enzyme reactions and has an essential role in the immune system.
ZINC	A cofactor for numerous enzyme reactions and directly or indirectly involved in supporting major metabolic pathways. Vital for growth, repair, and reproductive and immune health.
IODINE	An essential component of the thyroid hormones, which regulate metabolic rate, and of physical and mental development.
COPPER	Needed to produce red and white blood cells. Important for immune system support, bone health and brain development.
SELENIUM	A component of antioxidant enzymes, which help protect the body against oxidative damage. Vital for reproductive function, immune health and thyroid hormone production.
MANGANESE	Essential for bone formation and energy metabolism.

Other minerals include molybdenum, fluoride, boron, chromium, cobalt, sulphur, chloride, silicon and vanadium. These are needed in trace amounts and are plentiful in a balanced vegan diet.

SOURCES

Legumes, sesame seeds, tahini, green leafy vegetables like broccoli, cabbage and okra (not spinach), fortified milks, calcium-set tofu (look for calcium sulphate in the ingredients), dried fruit such as prunes, raisins, figs and apricots.

Beans, lentils, nuts, sunflower seeds and grains (especially oats).

Dark green leafy vegetables, avocados, cashews, almonds, Brazil nuts, beans, lentils, wholegrains, dark chocolate (cacao).

Table salt, salted nuts, miso, soy sauce (processed foods also often contain high amounts of sodium).

White beans, potatoes and sweet potatoes, beetroots, parsnips, spinach and bananas.

Green leafy vegetables, beans and lentils, tofu, chia, flax, hemp and pumpkin seeds, dried fruit, cashews, quinoa, amaranth and blackstrap molasses.

Beans and lentils, tofu, walnuts, cashews, chia, flax, hemp and pumpkin seeds, wholemeal bread, quinoa and wholegrains.

Sea vegetables, iodized salt and potatoes.

Seeds and nuts, wholegrains, dried beans and mushrooms.

Brazil nuts, kidney beans, yeast and wholegrains. Just one Brazil nut a day may meet your needs.

Wholegrains and cereals, kale, spinach, oatmeal, nuts, seeds and pineapples.

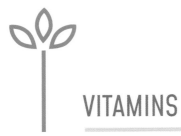

VITAMINS

Vitamins are organic compounds which are essential and are required by the body in small amounts. The vegan diet tends to provide good amounts of most vitamins, however special attention must be paid to two: vitamin B_{12} and vitamin D.

VITAMIN B_{12}

Since no plant food contains reliable amounts of vitamin B_{12}, it is particularly important for vegans to focus on sourcing and consuming this vital nutrient. This vitamin isn't made by plants nor animals, it's made by bacteria. Humans used to get this vitamin from foods which were contaminated with bacteria that had produced vitamin B_{12}, such as vegetables with miniscule traces of soil on them. However, these days our food is scrubbed clean and sterilized, so it is harder to source. We only need tiny amounts of this vitamin, and many foods are fortified with B_{12}, but vegans can still become deficient if they are not careful, with symptoms – such as pale skin, muscle weakness and numbing or tingling in the fingers – sometimes being slow to develop or intensifying over time. Luckily, deficiency isn't common, but it can be serious and can cause anemia and irreversible nerve damage. Supplementation is key.

VITAMIN D

Vitamin D deficiency in both vegans and non-vegans is relatively common. In fact, it is estimated that a staggering 1 billion people worldwide have vitamin D deficiency or insufficiency. Vitamin D isn't actually a vitamin at all – it is a pro-hormone produced from a reaction to UVA and UVB light (i.e. the glorious sunshine!). However, our modern lifestyles have resulted in less exposure to sunlight. Also, many of us live in northern latitudes which lack year-round sunshine, and when the sun does show its face, we (justifiably) slather sunscreen on, further blocking the production of vitamin D.

All of this means many people need to get vitamin D from their diet, and vegans can struggle with this as the limited sources, such as oily fish and eggs, are mainly animal based. In the UK it is recommended that all individuals, vegan or not, take a vitamin D supplement in the darker autumn and winter months to avoid deficiency. It may also be a good idea to get your vitamin D levels tested – ask your doctor for a 25-hydroxy test. This will help establish the right dose for you to supplement with.

Take vitamin D_3 supplements, not D_2. Vitamin D_3 is much more easily absorbed, however it isn't typically vegan, so be sure to find a supplement that is lichen-derived D_3.

tip

To improve vitamin D absorption, consume fortified foods and supplements with food that contains a little healthy fat (vitamin D is a fat-soluble vitamin).

Essential vitamins and where to find them

VITAMIN	FUNCTIONS	SOURCES
VITAMIN A	Essential to the normal function of the skin and mucous membranes such as the eyes, lungs and digestive system.	Dark green leafy vegetables as well as orange coloured fruit and vegetables such as carrots, mangoes, apricots and sweet potatoes.
VITAMIN C	Necessary for the growth, development and repair of all body tissues. Plays supportive roles in the immune system, wound healing, maintenance of cartilage, bones, teeth and skin.	Fruits such as oranges, kiwis, lemons, guava, grapefruits and strawberries, and vegetables such as broccoli, cauliflower, Brussels sprouts and sweet (bell) peppers.
VITAMIN D	Essential in bone health, and plays supportive roles in muscle functions and immune health.	The best source is the sunshine. Just 15–20 minutes on your face and arms daily should be enough (be sure to practice safe sun exposure). Some mushrooms may contain a little vitamin D (see page 62).
VITAMIN E	An antioxidant that protects cells against oxidative damage from free radicals.	Avocados, nuts such as almonds, Brazil nuts, hazelnuts and pine nuts, peanuts, seeds, Swiss chard, spinach and mangoes.
VITAMIN K	Plays an important role in blood clotting, bone metabolism and regulating blood calcium levels.	All green vegetables, prunes and kiwis.
B VITAMINS*	The B vitamins are collectively known as 'B-complex' vitamins, as they often work together in the body. They are known as the 'energy vitamins' as they play a major role in energy metabolism and the conversion of food into energy. They are also involved in many body functions such as cell, skin, bone, muscle and nervous system health.	Mushrooms, wholegrains, wheat germ, legumes, soya beans, walnuts, green leafy vegetables, sea greens, avocados, kelp and broccoli.

*(thiamine, riboflavin, niacin, pantothenic acid, biotin, vitamin B_6, vitamin B_{12} and folate).

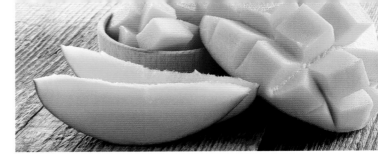

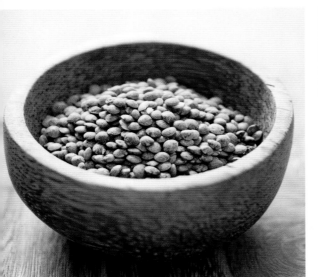

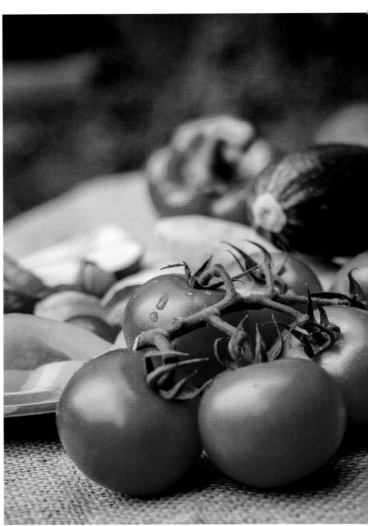

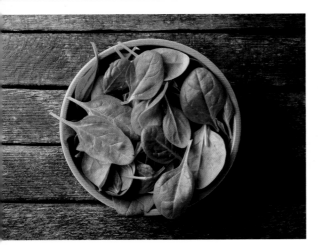

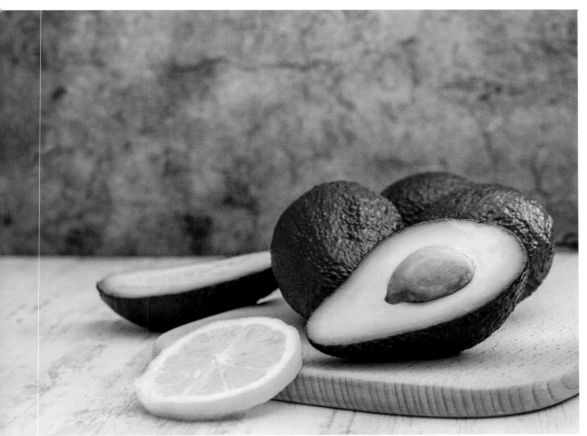

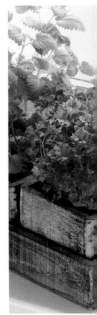

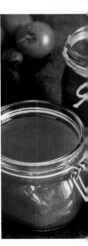

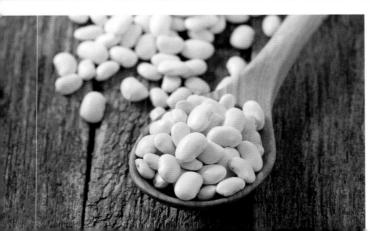

DO I NEED TO TAKE SUPPLEMENTS?

When it comes to maintaining good health, a well-balanced diet is key. However, sometimes food alone cannot provide us with all the nutrients we need.

This could be due to the way food is produced, such as the use of highly intensive agricultural farming techniques, which can deplete the soil of essential nutrients, leading to lower levels of nutrients in our food. Some studies have suggested that compared to the fruits and vegetables of our great grandparent's times, today's crops contain less magnesium, zinc, vitamins A, C and E, calcium, iron and potassium, and have reduced quantities of other nutrients such as Vitamin B_2 and protein.

At the same time, another symptom of our modern lifestyles is a significant increase in exposure to pesticides, stress, environmental pollution, highly processed foods and medication use.

These aspects of modern life – the potential decrease in nutrients from our food (and therefore possible deficiency) coupled with an increased need for them – can undoubtedly increase our individual need for extra nutrients to support our health. We may well be consuming enough to 'tick over', but there's a big difference between that and feeling your best! Therefore, even if you do eat a reasonably healthy diet, it may be useful to include a good daily multivitamin and mineral supplement in your diet to bridge the gap.

VEGAN-SPECIFIC SUPPLEMENTS

As a vegan, daily vitamin-B_{12} supplementation is non-negotiable: you simply can't get enough from your food, on a regular basis, to meet your needs. Vitamin D supplementation is also strongly recommended during the darker winter months (see page 36). An algae-derived omega-3 supplement (in the form of EPA/DHA) may also be a good addition if your diet doesn't contain significant amounts of this nutrient from food sources (see pages 27). Furthermore, as vegans can have significantly lower levels of iodine in their diets, it may be a good idea to supplement with this, too. A good multivitamin and mineral supplement may contain enough B_{12}, vitamin D and iodine in the doses that are right for you. However, before supplementing with iodine as a standalone supplement (i.e. not in a multivitamin/mineral), do speak to a dietitian or registered nutritionist as too much iodine can have detrimental effects on your health.

Important:

Nutrients can be powerful. Always consult with your doctor before starting any supplementations, especially if you are on any medication, have medical concerns or if you are pregnant and/or breastfeeding. Stop immediately if you feel any side effects and review your supplement regime every six months.

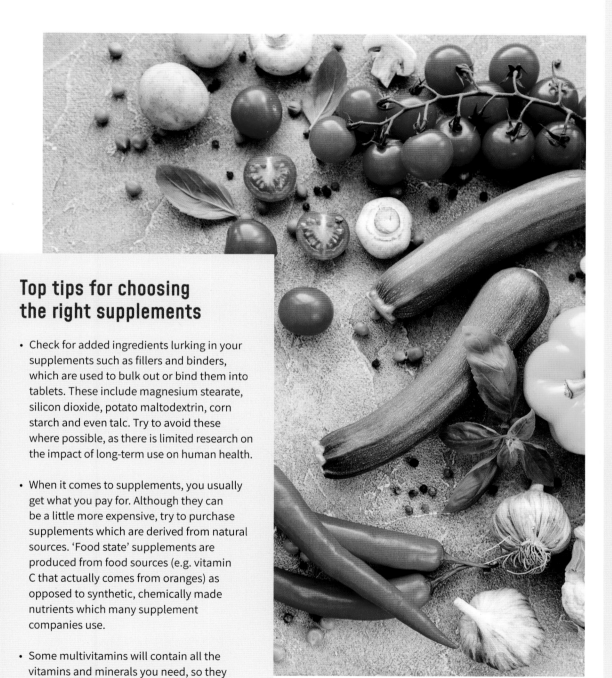

Top tips for choosing the right supplements

- Check for added ingredients lurking in your supplements such as fillers and binders, which are used to bulk out or bind them into tablets. These include magnesium stearate, silicon dioxide, potato maltodextrin, corn starch and even talc. Try to avoid these where possible, as there is limited research on the impact of long-term use on human health.

- When it comes to supplements, you usually get what you pay for. Although they can be a little more expensive, try to purchase supplements which are derived from natural sources. 'Food state' supplements are produced from food sources (e.g. vitamin C that actually comes from oranges) as opposed to synthetic, chemically made nutrients which many supplement companies use.

- Some multivitamins will contain all the vitamins and minerals you need, so they may be a good option to consider.

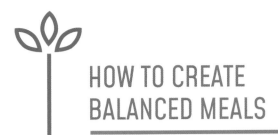

HOW TO CREATE BALANCED MEALS

It can be easy to fall into the trap of creating meals that are unbalanced by having big plates of pasta most nights, or regularly substituting meat with highly processed foods.

When taking meat, dairy and eggs out of your diet, it's important to consider how to replace them in a healthy way. Many people find they actually eat a more varied diet and get quite inventive in the kitchen when they turn vegan, so get those creative juices flowing! Saying that, don't feel you need to spend hours cooking up complicated meals: simple good food made with fresh, whole ingredients is key. Of course, you can have your cake and eat it too, but perhaps not every day.

tip

Keep hydrated by drinking eight glasses of water a day.

Aim to drink it away from mealtimes as too much water drunk with food can dilute digestive enzymes and have a negative impact on digestion. Do, however, sip some water with meals.

Fact:

We all know we should eat our greens, but how about blues, yellows, oranges and reds, too? Not only do all plants contain loads of vitamins, minerals and fibre, they also contain tiny little components that give them their colour.

This is where the magic happens, as every colour is a different set of healing chemicals known as *phytonutrients* – 25,000 different phytonutrients can be found in plant foods such as fruit, vegetables, pulses, spices and herbs. These phytonutrients have a remarkable ability to protect against inflammation and chronic disease.

FAT IS YOUR FRIEND

Consuming a little healthy fat with your meals, perhaps drizzling a little extra virgin olive oil over your vegetables, or sprinkling seeds over fruit, can help your body absorb certain antioxidants and phytonutrients. Fats also help you absorb the fat-soluble vitamins A, D, E and K.

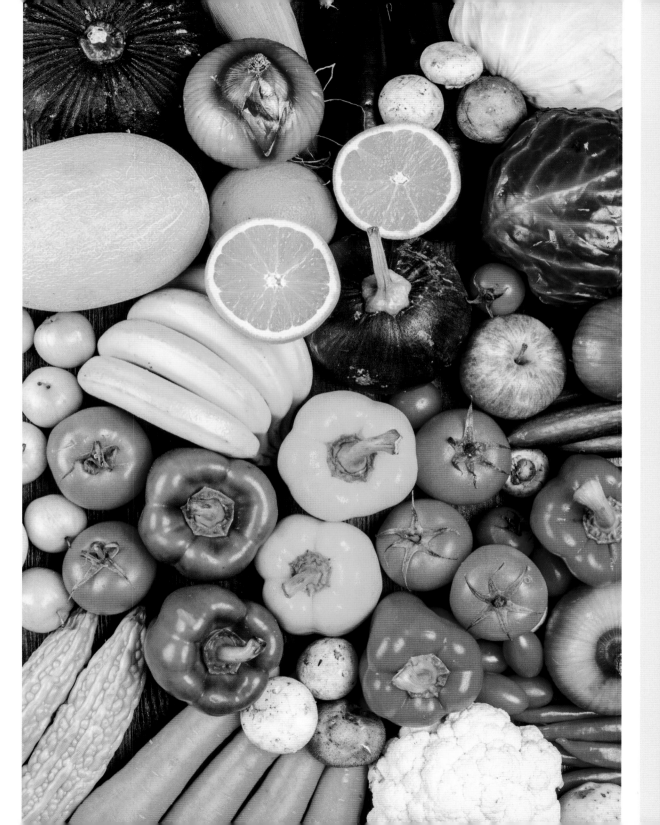

Perfect portions

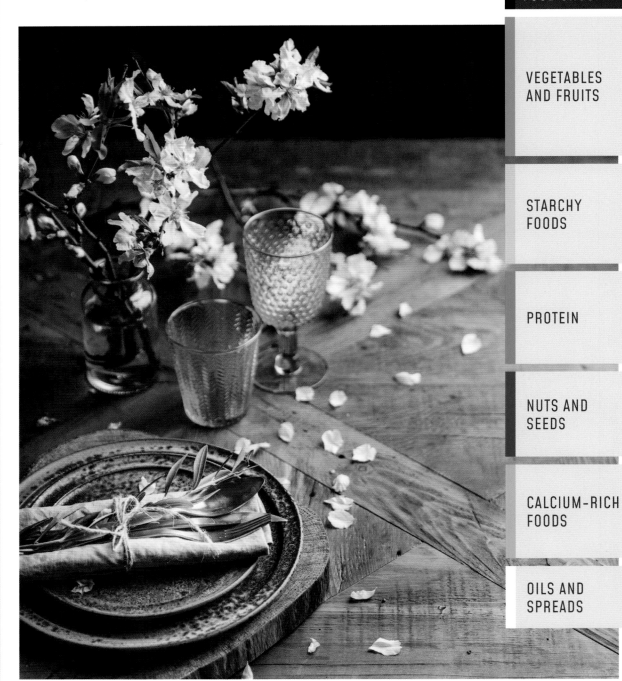

VEGETABLES
AND FRUITS

STARCHY
FOODS

PROTEIN

NUTS AND
SEEDS

CALCIUM-RICH
FOODS

OILS AND
SPREADS

PORTION SIZE

Aim to eat a rainbow of colours throughout the day: five 80g (3oz) portions composing of two pieces of fruit and at least three portions of veggies. Make vegetables the main event in a dish – they should fill half your plate. Aim to have at least one portion of green leafy greens per day.

Include one portion at each meal. A portion size would be the size of your clenched fist (roughly 3 tablespoons) - and should fill no more than a quarter of your plate.

Aim to have a portion at each meal. The portion size should be roughly the size of the palm of your hand or a quarter of your plate of food.

1 cupped handful daily, as a snack or as part of a meal.

Ensure you are consuming plenty of calcium-rich foods daily.

Use 1 tablespoon with each meal.

SOURCES

An 80g (3oz) portion of vegetables would be two broccoli spears or 3 heaped tablespoons of cooked vegetables such as carrots, peas or sweetcorn. An 80g (3oz) portion of fruit could be a thick slice of watermelon, a whole piece of fruit such as an apple or orange, or two smaller fruits such as a couple of plums. Dried fruit should be a 30g (1oz) portion. Potatoes don't count in this category, as they are considered a starchy component of a meal.

Brown rice or wholegrain pasta, potatoes, sweet potatoes, oats, wholemeal bread, quinoa and cereals. Always opt for whole grains over refined grains. You could include sprouted grains here, too.

Tofu, beans and pulses in any form. For example, a bean burger, lentil dhal or soup, bean or lentil salads, roasted chickpeas, sautéed tofu or tempeh, or soya alternatives to milk and yoghurt.

Aim to consume nuts and seeds that are particularly high in omega-3 fats such as flax, hemp, chia, walnuts, or 1 tablespoon of walnut oil. Other nuts/seeds are also important, such as Brazil nuts, cashews and almonds.

Leafy vegetables, tahini, fortified milks and yoghurts, dried figs and almonds. 100g (3½oz) of calcium-set tofu will provide roughly half the recommended daily allowance. 400ml (14fl oz) of fortified plant milk can provide about two-thirds of the recommended daily allowance.

Plant-based spreads (always look for 'non-hydrogenated' on the label to avoid trans fats), rapeseed and olive oils, and cooking oils.

Your vegan pantry

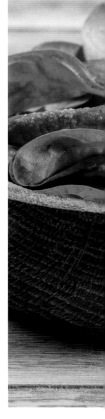
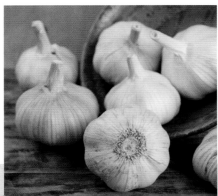
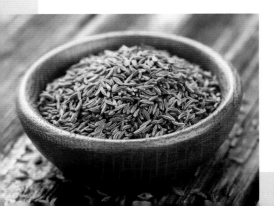
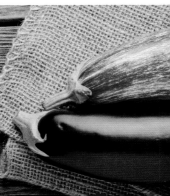

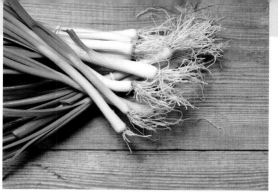

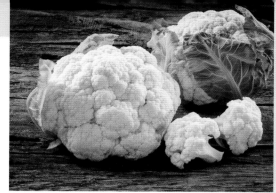

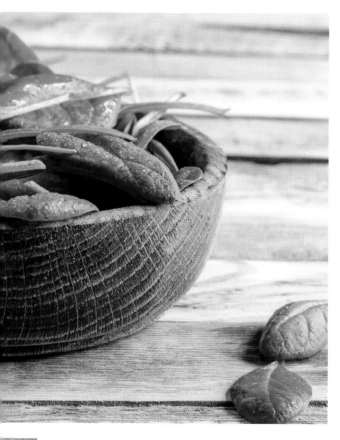

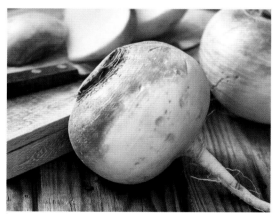

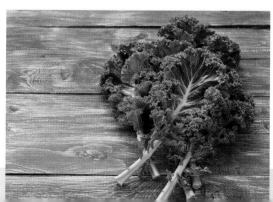

Tubers & ROOT VEGETABLES

Fibrous root vegetables have long been recognized as a winter staple, even a year-round one. Colourful in their many forms, they are nutritionally rich and at their best in winter months through to spring. The smallest root vegetables tend to be the most tender, and some can be eaten both raw and cooked.

Their vitamin content decreases the longer they are out of the ground – eat them while they are fresh and firm and scrub root vegetables instead of peeling them, if you can, as most of the flavour sits just under the skin (except with turnips and celeriac).

POTATOES

This starchy tuber hails from South America. It was introduced to Europe in the sixteenth century by returning Spanish explorers and is now a staple food that is cultivated the world over (there are more than 200 species). The potato belongs to the deadly nightshade plant family, the same family as the tomato and pepper, and is a good source of complex carbohydrates, dietary fibre, protein and essential minerals. Crops are largely divided into three categories: all-purpose/all-rounders, waxy and floury. Small, early-cropping varieties, such as the sweet and buttery Jersey Royals, are referred to as 'new' potatoes and they hold together better during cooking than floury varieties, which have a fluffy texture and suit frying, roasting and baking. The mild flavour of potatoes – they contain about 80 per cent water – makes them a versatile ingredient. Keep them in a dark, cool place, but not the fridge, and avoid any that develop a green tinge.

NUTRITIONAL BENEFITS
Rich in vitamin C and potassium, and a good source of folate, fibre (when cooked with skin on) and iron. They also contain vitamin B_1 (thiamine).

SERVING SUGGESTIONS
Steam or boil waxy potatoes, or roast them in their skins and serve them with a spiced tomato sauce; make potato gnocchi by binding baked floury potato flesh with flour then boiling; cut floury potatoes into wedges or chips, par-boil, then toss in oil and roast; steam or boil Jersey Royals and serve with asparagus; bake new potatoes in parchment with garlic, oil and fresh herbs; roast potatoes with lemon and oregano; make a potato curry southern Indian style with curry leaves, coconut milk, tomato and warm spices; top flatbread or pizza with thinly sliced new potatoes before baking; make a chunky potato soup with onion, carrot and celery and add small pasta shapes.

PARSNIPS

The parsnip is native to Central and southern Europe and has been cultivated since ancient times to produce edible roots. Before the arrival of the potato in Europe it was an important staple food and a major source of starch in winter months. In medieval times it was also used as a sugar substitute, by crushing the root to draw off the juice, then boiling the juice down to a syrup, but once sugar was available its popularity waned and in much of southern Europe it had to make do with being used primarily as cattle fodder. Parsnips have a sweet, nutty flavour, and those harvested in winter are said to be the sweetest, as exposure to frost increases the plant's conversion of starch to sugar. Spices work particularly well with the sweetness and earthiness of the flesh. If your parsnips have been hanging around the vegetable drawer a little too long, remove the core before cooking them, as it can be tough and woody.

NUTRITIONAL BENEFITS

Richer in most vitamins and minerals than carrots, and a good source of potassium, phosphorus, folic acid, calcium and magnesium.

SERVING SUGGESTIONS

Quarter and par-boil parsnips then toss in maple syrup and oil (and a sprinkle of Chinese 5-spice or smoked paprika, if you like) before roasting; pare into long strips with a vegetable peeler and deep-fry in sunflower oil; make a spiced parsnip soup with cumin, coriander, onions and vegetable stock, roasting the parsnips first; make parsnip mash, adding a little grated nutmeg to serve.

CARROTS

The large carrot we're familiar with descended from a small, wild, bitter carrot which had pale or purple flesh; they only acquired their orange tinge in the sixteenth or seventeenth century when Holland developed a hybrid variety. They vary widely in size, from long and tapered to round or finger-sized, and in colour, they vary from purple and yellow to orange, white and dark red. Spring carrots

are the most tender and sweetest, and heritage varieties have a complex flavour that their maincrop orange counterparts rarely retain. They are eaten raw or cooked, and in Asia are often preserved in syrups and jams.

NUTRITIONAL BENEFITS

Rich in carotenoids and vitamin A, and vitamins B_3, C and E. Eaten raw, they provide potassium, calcium, iron and zinc, but these nutrients are diminished during cooking.

SERVING SUGGESTIONS

Make carrot juice, adding ginger and orange juice; grate for a carrot cake, adding grated courgette and a little mixed spice; roast and serve with a green herb and hazelnut pesto or gremolata; make hummus with roasted carrots and tahini instead of chickpeas; scrub, grate and mix with grated beetroot, lemon zest, coriander and olive oil for a bright, fluorescent salad; par-boil, then cook in an orange-juice glaze with vegan butter and caraway seeds or tarragon; slice and pickle with dill seeds, fennel seeds or bay; toss grated carrot through a cold Asian noodle salad with edamame beans; make a carrot dhal with turmeric and curry leaves.

tip

Remove and discard the leafy tops before storing, as they draw moisture from the roots.

SWEET POTATOES

Native to tropical America, this tuberous root from the morning glory family was introduced to Europe over 300 years ago. White and yellow-fleshed varieties are particularly popular in tropical regions (where it is a staple crop) and orange-fleshed varieties most common in the US. Yellow or orange-fleshed sweet potatoes are a richer source of carotene (a source of vitamin A) than the white variety, yet all shapes and colours of sweet potato are highly nutritious. It is unrelated to the ordinary potato and is sometimes confused with the yam, which has a similar shape. The creamy and moist flesh is nutrient-dense and high in starch, though lower in protein than potatoes. Their honey sweetness is further heightened by maple syrup or brown sugar at Thanksgiving in the US, and in Asia they are roasted by street vendors. Store at room temperature, not in the fridge.

NUTRITIONAL BENEFITS
Rich in calcium, magnesium, potassium, folic acid, vitamins C and E, phosphorus and beta-carotene.

SERVING SUGGESTIONS
Cut into wedges and fry to make chips; bake like jacket potatoes; make a sweet potato mac 'n' cheese with a vegan béchamel; bake a whole sweet potato, then peel, mash and combine with flour and ground cinnamon to make gnocchi; combine roasted chunks of sweet potato with warm spices and herbs or spinach and bake in vegan pastry to make a pasty (or filo to make samosas); combine with red lentils to make a warming dhal; use slices as a layer in a vegan lasagne.

TURNIPS

This underrated member of the cabbage family, commonly confused with the larger swede, has been widely cultivated for over 4,000 years and is one of the oldest European food crops. It is technically the swollen lower stem and upper part of the taproot of a brassica, but is sold as a root vegetable.

Turnips vary in size widely and range from purple to white to yellow in colour, though most are white-fleshed (often with a scarlet or purple-tinged collar). The smaller (younger) the turnip, the sweeter its flesh. The pungent, leafy tops are extremely nutritious and rich in folic acid and calcium. If you can buy turnips with their tops intact, eat the tops as soon as possible. A variety of turnip is grown in Italy specifically for its edible bitter greens, known as *cime di rapa*. To soften any bitterness in the flesh, peel and cook until just tender before serving. The youngest white turnips can be eaten raw and have a crisp, peppery and nutty taste.

NUTRITIONAL BENEFITS
Rich in vitamin C, calcium, magnesium, phosphorus, potassium and folic acid.

SERVING SUGGESTIONS
Roast young whole turnips with apple and onion; braise or mash with carrots; quarter and pickle with white wine or cider vinegar, salt and garlic, adding beetroot if you want to give the pickle a pink colour; braise turnip tops in oil with chilli; make a turnip kimchi with Korean chilli flakes, garlic and ginger; peel, blanch to remove bitterness, then roast whole; cube, roast and stir through a risotto.

CELERIAC

Also known as celery root, this swollen stem base is closely related to celery and isn't strictly a root vegetable (what botanical category it sits under remains a matter of debate). It derives from wild celery native to Europe and the Middle East, and its flavour resembles both parsley and celery. Under its gnarly, unprepossessing exterior sits sweet, pale flesh. Its delicate nuttiness is appealing raw and becomes sweeter on cooking. Use a sharp, robust knife

tip

The flesh of celeriac discolours quickly, so place it in acidulated water (water with added lemon juice) if not eating it straight away.

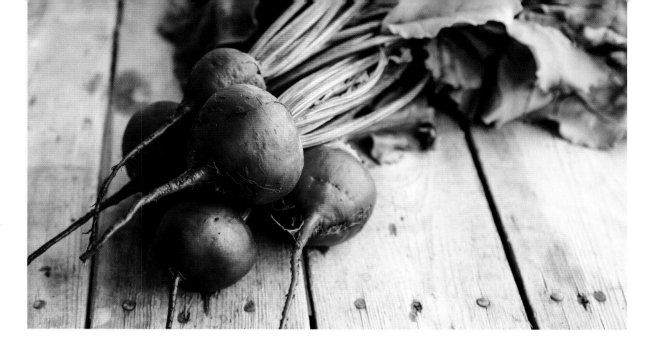

rather than a vegetable peeler to prepare it: it takes effort to remove the bark-like skin. Adding a good-quality fat to a celeriac dish helps boost the absorption of its vitamins.

NUTRITIONAL BENEFITS
Rich in calcium, magnesium, potassium, vitamins K and C, and B vitamins.

SERVING SUGGESTIONS
Cut into matchsticks and combine with a mustard-rich dressing – raw apple adds a lovely tartness, too; cube and boil until soft, then drain and blitz to a mash; combine celeriac mash with mashed potato or cooked apple; make celeriac and celery soup with a little onion and leek; cut celeriac into ribbons, blanch and serve with a sauce as an alternative to pasta; roasted whole, drizzle with olive oil or salt-bake.

BEETROOTS

Beetroot – descended from wild sea beetroot – has been cultivated and enjoyed since Roman times, though the globular beetroot we're familiar with was not developed until the sixteenth century. Grown widely in temperate climates around the world, particularly Europe and America, common beetroot is red, but others are cultivated for eating too, including striped Chioggia and golden beetroot. Its firm, juicy flesh has a robust and earthy flavour that sweetens on cooking (particularly roasting). The iron-rich leaves are edible, and have a similar taste to chard (which is from the same plant family – see page 75) or spinach. Cook leaves and stems separately, as the stems need a longer cooking time.

NUTRITIONAL BENEFITS
Rich in calcium, magnesium, iron, phosphorus, potassium, manganese, folic acid and vitamin C.

SERVING SUGGESTIONS
Make a soup with ginger, orange, onion and beetroot; sauté beetroot tops with garlic and oil and top with toasted walnuts; roast wedges of beetroot in oil with caraway seeds; add juiced beetroot to a tart, mustardy dressing; deep-fry thin strips in sunflower oil; make an Iranian beetroot borani, substituting yoghurt for vegan yoghurt; cook until tender, then slice and bake with puff pastry and thyme to make a savoury tarte tatin; grate for a salad and dress with a coconut yoghurt dressing; combine grated beetroot and apple with watercress and a lemony dressing; grate it raw into the batter for a dark chocolate cake or brownies.

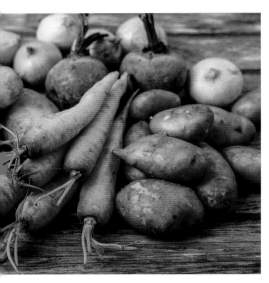

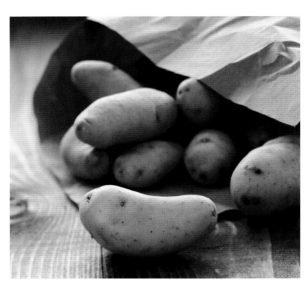

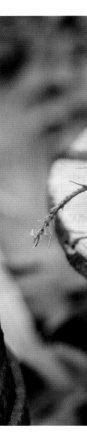

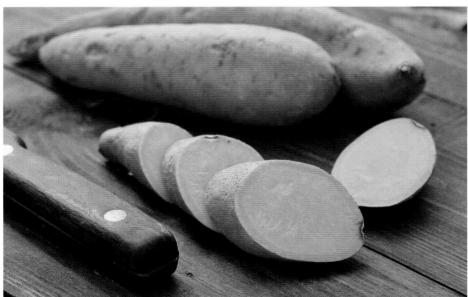

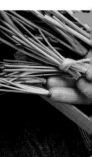

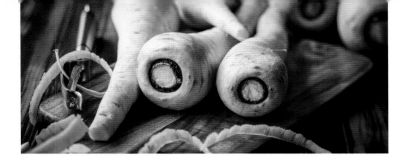

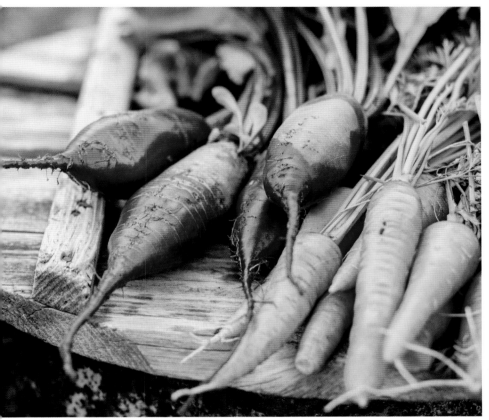

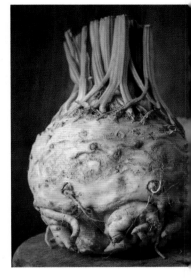

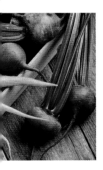

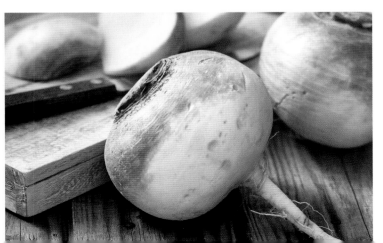

Cucumbers
SQUASHES & GOURDS

Cucumber, squashes and gourds belong to the plant genus Cucurbita and are vine-growing fruit, not vegetables. Courgettes and marrows are largely native to the Americas and grow in warm, temperate climates. They contain a large amount of water (around 90 per cent or higher) and their key nutritional asset is the carotenes in deep yellow and orange-fleshed varieties.

Squash are available in a colourful range of shapes and sizes, making for a show like no other in autumn greengrocer displays. They are typically split into two types: summer and winter. Summer squash, such as courgettes, are immature fruit with a thin edible skin and soft, pale mild-flavoured flesh and winter squash, such as pumpkins and acorn squash, are the weightier mature fruits, with tougher skin, firm, mealy flesh and a more robust, sweet flavour. Many winter squashes are rich in beta-carotene and other carotenoids, as well as starch. The mild flavour of most Cucurbita makes them suitable for both sweet and savoury dishes.

The delicate flowers of courgette, squashes, pumpkins and marrows can all be battered and fried.

CUCUMBERS

Said to be native to the Himalayas, cucumber has been cultivated for as long as 3,000 years and was adored by the ancient Egyptians, Greeks and Romans. It arrived in Britain around the end of the sixteenth century and was bred over the centuries to lose the natural bitterness of its ancestors. Like the melons to which they are related, the flesh is refreshing, juicy and crisp – modern cultivars contain about 96 per cent water. The most common variety is long, with a smooth, dark green skin, but there are also fatter ridged cucumbers (which must be peeled before eating), and short stubby cucumbers that are used for pickling. Press the stalk end of a cucumber to check for freshness – it should be firm. Avoid peeling the common, smooth-skinned cucumber as the skin contains most of the cucumber's nutrients. They can be eaten raw, pickled or cooked. To intensify the cucumber flavour, halve, remove the watery core, then slice or grate the flesh and place the cucumber in a bowl with a pinch of salt. Toss and set aside for about 20 minutes in a sieve, to draw out some of the water.

NUTRITIONAL BENEFITS
They contain potassium and a small amount of vitamin C: unpeeled they contain some carotenes.

SERVING SUGGESTIONS
Cut ribbons of cucumber, salt and drain, then pickle with white wine or cider vinegar, salt, sugar and coriander seeds or dill (or both); make a cooling cucumber and mint granita; chop and stir through freekeh salad or cold Japanese rice bowl; blitz cucumber with lettuce and herbs to make a chilled soup; add to a gazpacho; make the Sichuan dish of smashed ('smacked') cucumber by bashing cucumber with a rolling pin until broken into bite-sized pieces, then salt and drain, before combining with a sweet-sour dressing; add slices to

iced water with a grind of black pepper to make a refreshing drink; dice and add to a Middle Eastern fattoush salad.

COURGETTES

Italian plant breeders developed the thin-skinned courgette (known as zucchini in the US and Italy), a type of summer squash, in the early 1900s. These immature, tender marrows mature in mid-summer and have a smooth, green, striped or yellow edible skin, and a mild, delicate taste. Choose small, firm courgettes for the best flavour – they are at their best when they are 12–15cm long. Smaller, subtly nutty courgettes can be eaten in their entirety, but larger ones should be topped and tailed. They have a high water content, so avoid steaming or boiling them as this can make them mushy. Courgette flowers can be deep-fried.

NUTRITIONAL BENEFITS
A good source of B vitamins, potassium and vitamins C and K.

SERVING SUGGESTIONS
Make courgette fritti by cutting courgettes into thin strips, soaking them in vegan milk, then tossing them in seasoned flour before deep-frying; braise with good-quality oil and dill; add to a spiced vegetable laksa or vegetable lasagne; chargrill thick courgette ribbons and combine with cooked beans or grains and a punchy herb and lemon dressing; add to a ratatouille; shave raw into a salad; lightly braise and serve with fresh chopped herbs and a drizzle of oil; make a Provencal-style courgette and tomato gratin; add grilled slices to a summer vegetable pilaf; grate into savoury muffin batter; deep-fry courgette flowers, removing the stamen first; bake sliced courgettes and tomatoes with oregano, topped with grated vegan cheese.

PUMPKINS

The best known of the winter squash, pumpkins have been cultivated since ancient times in Europe, the Middle East and the Americas. They are a traditional ingredient in US Thanksgiving celebrations, which would not be complete without a spiced pumpkin pie (made with tinned pumpkin purée), but in the UK they are better known for carving into ghoulish Halloween faces than for their culinary virtues. Under the tough skin sits lightly sweet, deep orange flesh. Buy them whole rather than cut, as once a pumpkin is sliced it loses much of its flavour, and go for small pumpkins for cooking, as the flesh of larger ones can be unpleasantly mealy. Carbohydrates are more concentrated in pumpkins and other winter squash than in summer squash.

NUTRITIONAL BENEFITS
The flesh is rich in beta-carotene and the seeds are a good source of iron, protein, oil and a range of minerals including potassium, copper and zinc.

SERVING SUGGESTIONS
Roast or stew (with garlic and onions if making a savoury dish), then use the cooked flesh to fill savoury pasta, purée with stock and spices to make a velvety, rich soup, or sweeten with cinnamon and sugar and use as a filling for sweet ravioli; slice and layer with onions then bake in the oven; roast halved and deseeded, then scoop out the flesh and stir into risotto; separate the seeds from the woolly pulp, season, toss in oil and roast to eat as a snack (the edible inner kernels contain nutritious oils); make pumpkin seed butter by blitzing seed kernels with a neutral oil and salt.

BUTTERNUT SQUASHES

Originating from Guatemala and Mexico, this common variety of winter squash has a pale, smooth skin, bulbous base and dense, orange flesh and is available all year round. It is easier to prepare than most squash varieties, as the skin is thinner. The firm flesh becomes sweet and nutty when cooked, avoiding the tendency of other winter squash to be too watery or floury. It also holds its shape well in curries and vegetable stews.

NUTRITIONAL BENEFITS
Particularly rich in carotenoids (similar levels as sweet potatoes and apricots), and a good source of calcium, magnesium, phosphorus, potassium and vitamin C.

SERVING SUGGESTIONS
Dice, roast and use in a South Indian curry; grate and combine with sautéed onion, garlic, toasted spices or herbs, breadcrumbs and vegan cheese to make polpette, then shallow fry; make a Moroccan squash and chickpea stew; add roasted squash to a spelt risotto; make a squash and lentil soup; dice and roast with oil, chilli flakes and garlic; deep-fry squash skin peelings to make nutritious crisps.

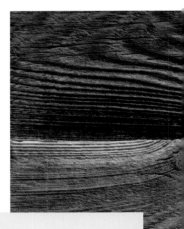

Other squashes & gourds

PATTY PAN: This white, pale green or yellow summer squash has scalloped edges and a delicate flavour similar to courgettes (but firmer textured flesh). Boil or steam whole until tender. They are best eaten when about 10cm in diameter.

MARROW: A large, mature version of courgette. Avoid huge ones, which will have lost their sweet freshness. Hollow out, stuff and bake, or use to make a spiced chutney.

BOTTLE GOURD: This tropical variety of winter squash has a nutty flavour and holds its shape well in cooking.

WINTER MELON: This large Asian vegetable resembles a courgette and has a similar delicate, mild taste. Also known as 'fuzzy melon', the skin is covered in tiny hairs. It should be cooked before eating. In China, it is used as an edible container for soup.

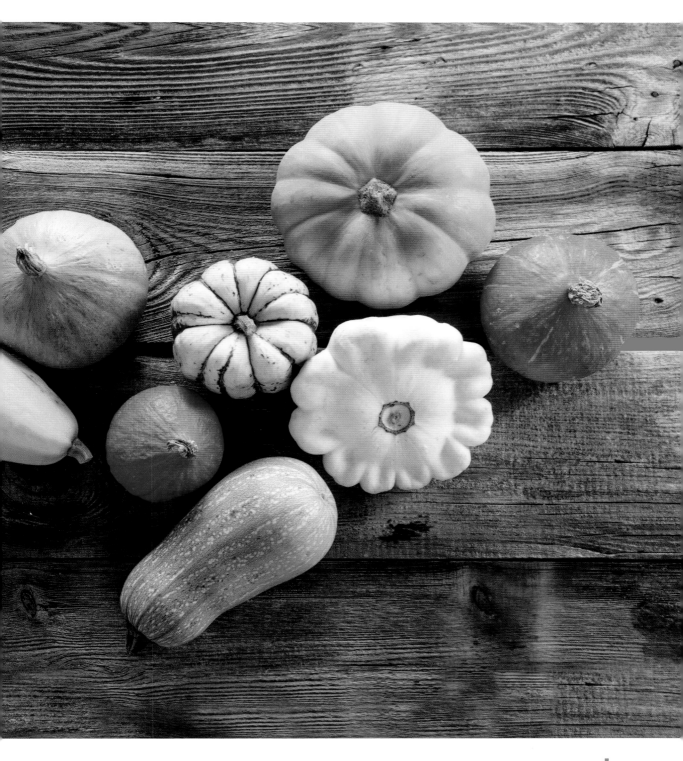

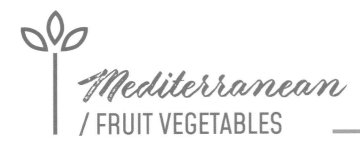

Mediterranean
/ FRUIT VEGETABLES

These fleshy fruiting vegetables originate from tropical and sub-tropical regions and are available in a vivid array of colours. Their bright and vibrant pigments indicate their high nutrient value, and all three complement each other, whether slow-roasted, sautéed or grilled.

TOMATOES

This fruit of the vegetable world comes from a tropical plant native to the Americas. It was brought to Europe by Spanish explorers in the early sixteenth century and is now cultivated worldwide, particularly in the Mediterranean, where it is a key culinary ingredient. Through domestication, the bitterness of its ancestors was bred out and their intense, sweet-sharp flavour became predominant. Varieties number in their thousands, and range from sweet cherry tomatoes to large, fleshy beefsteak and specialist heritage tomatoes. A sun-ripened summer tomato has a vastly superior taste than the fridge-cold hot-house tomatoes available through colder months. Unripe green tomatoes (not to be confused with heritage green varieties) are used in pickles and preserves.

The lycopene in tomatoes is best absorbed by the body when tomatoes are cooked in oil (or eaten with avocado) and it's found in high concentrations in tomato paste. Tomato flavour can be intensified by a touch of sugar and acidic ingredients such as vinegar and lemon juice. Store at room temperature.

NUTRITIONAL BENEFITS
Rich in the carotenoid lycopene, beta-carotene, and vitamins C and E. Also contains calcium, magnesium, phosphorus and folic acid.

SERVING SUGGESTIONS
Blitz to make a refreshing cold tomato soup, such as a gazpacho, made with bread, tomatoes, cucumber, sweet peppers, garlic, vinegar and oil; when making a tomato sauce, add a tomato vine too, if you have it, to deepen and intensify the tomato flavour; use overripe tomatoes to make sauces or rub onto toasted bread with garlic; make a tomato and basil granita; slice and bake with herbs and caramelized onion on a puff pastry base; make a Tuscan bread and tomato salad (panzanella) with ciabatta, tomatoes, oil, vinegar, garlic, capers and herbs; roast cherry tomatoes on the vine; to remove tomato skin, cut a small cross in the base, place in boiling water for 30 seconds, then drain, refresh in cold water and peel; make American fried green tomatoes by coating thickly sliced green tomatoes in flour, then whipped aquafaba and vegan milk, before frying; use roasted tomatoes to make tomato ketchup; slow-cook runner beans with chopped tomatoes and good olive oil; make a Mexican salsa or spiced chutney; add a pinch of ground clove to a tomato sauce to enhance the tomato flavour.

PEPPERS

Native to the tropical regions of the Americas, capsicums (sweet peppers) were brought to Europe by Spanish explorers in the sixteenth century. Also known as 'bell peppers' this hollow fruit is mild, not spicy, and can be eaten raw or cooked. It is one of the richest sources of red-coloured carotenoid pigment, lycopene, and contains more vitamin C than oranges (green peppers twice as much, red peppers four times as much). The difference in colour signifies ripeness and sweetness: green (unripe) peppers have a tart, grassy flavour, and ripe peppers (which range from red, yellow or orange to almost black) are sweet. They should be glossy and firm, and the bitter seeds and white membrane should be removed before eating. Long, tapered varieties such as Romano have a thinner skin and fuller sweet flavour than 'bell' peppers.

NUTRITIONAL BENEFITS
A rich source of beta-carotene and vitamins C, A and B_6.

SERVING SUGGESTIONS
To remove the skin, grill or roast until the skin blisters and blackens, then place in a bag to steam for a few minutes before rubbing away the skin; use roasted peppers to make a smoky hummus with chickpeas, romesco sauce, or a roasted red pepper soup made with tomatoes; slice fresh pepper and stew with onions and tomatoes to make an Italian peperonata; add to an oven-roasted ratatouille; stir-fry and add to tortilla wraps with other grilled vegetables, herbs, a vegan yoghurt and lime dressing and hot sauce; add strips of pepper to a vegetable stir-fry; stuff; use green or yellow peppers in a stir-fry; add diced red pepper to a vegetarian rice gumbo.

AUBERGINES

From the same plant family as tomatoes and potatoes, aubergines are thought to have originated in the Old World, going on to take root in tropical Asia. Arab traders introduced them to Spain and Africa in the Middle Ages, and from there they made it to the rest of Europe. They have become integral to Greek and Turkish cuisines, and in southern Asia, small, crunchy aubergines are used as a condiment and in curries. Aubergines can be large and round, elongated or egg-shaped and range from the size of a pea to the size of a football. The smooth, shiny edible skin varies in colour, but the most common variety is a deep purple. On cooking, the slightly bitter, spongy-textured flesh becomes meltingly soft and creamy. Store in a cool place, but not the fridge. Some recommend salting (degorging) aubergines before using, to remove bitterness, but in most modern varieties this characteristic has been bred out, so there is no need, though salting the cut flesh before cooking can help reduce its absorption of oil and make a dish less rich.

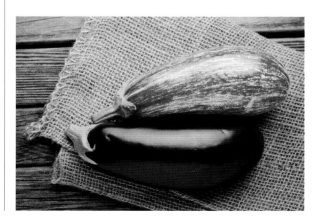

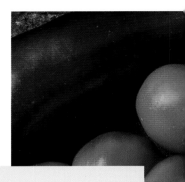

NUTRITIONAL BENEFITS
A good source of minerals, including potassium, and some carotenes.

SERVING SUGGESTIONS
Slowly flame-grill or roast aubergines whole, until the flesh softens and collapses, then make the Middle Eastern aubergine dip, baba ganoush, with lemon and oil (add garlic and tahini too, if you like); make an aubergine and tomato curry; halve aubergine lengthways, score the flesh in a criss-cross pattern, drizzle with oil and roast until soft, then baste with a miso and mirin dressing and grill until golden; make a sweet-sour caponata salad with aubergines and tomatoes; make a warm-spiced rice pilaf, then add roasted cubed aubergine and stir through some toasted pine nuts; cut into sticks and fry tempura-style in a light batter; make Moroccan aubergine and chickpeas stew; fry with green pepper to make the Turkish dish *patlican biber*.

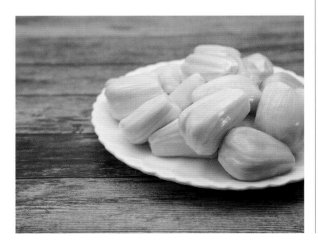

Jackfruit

Jackfruit is thought to be native to South India. The large, heavy fruit belongs to the same tropical plant family as breadfruit, and is a popular ingredient in Indian and Sri Lankan cuisines. Enclosed within green, knobbly skin are pods of potent yellow flesh with a spongy, stringy texture. (A red-fleshed, milder-flavoured jackfruit is also cultivated in India.) In its growing areas it is used prolifically as both a 'hard' (unripe) 'semi-hard' (semi-ripe) or 'soft' (ripe) fruit.

The flesh is typically cooked as a starchy, fibrous vegetable when unripe, in chutneys and pickles, biryani, curries, tacos, burritos, fritters and stews, and eaten as a soft fruit in desserts and preserves when ripe and sweet. Jackfruit is used in the west as a meat substitute in savoury dishes, and is a good source of protein, fibre, vitamins A and C, and minerals. Look out for fresh jackfruit in Asian shops, or used good-quality tinned jackfruit in water.

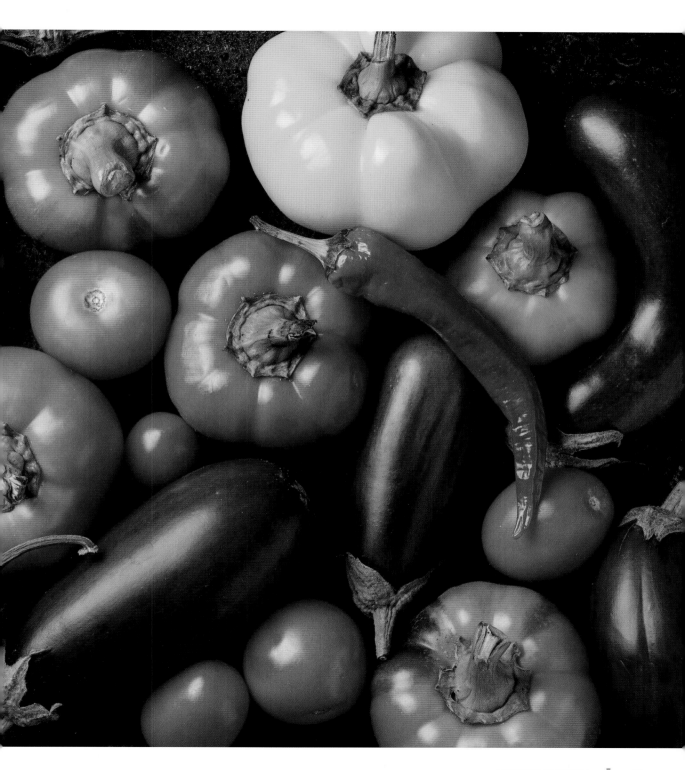

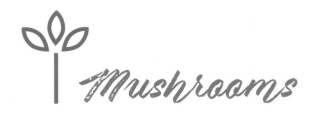

Mushrooms

Fungi grow in shaded, damp habitats such as forests, woods, meadows, and parklands throughout temperate regions, yet only a tiny fraction of the thousands of edible mushroom species have been successfully cultivated. With a few exceptions, mushrooms are harvested in early autumn and their characteristic earthy, umami flavour adds a savoury, vegetal note to food and a meaty texture. Wild mushrooms and shiitake are more intensely savoury than cultivated mushrooms. The three mushrooms opposite are the key cultivated mushroom – Agaricus bisporus – at its various stages of development. They should smell earthy and sweet – avoid using any that are moist or smell sour. The skin of mushroom caps contains much of the flavour, so avoid peeling them unless necessary.

Most mushrooms contain 80–90 per cent water, a range of minerals and B vitamins, vitamin D and a large amount of potassium.

Store mushrooms in paper bags rather than plastic, to avoid them becoming slimy, and wipe them clean with kitchen paper before using. If you wash them, use them immediately after, before they become soggy.

Quorn is a microfungus developed to have a similar texture to meat.

WHITE MUSHROOMS

The common mushroom accounts for over 50 per cent of the world mushroom production and it has been cultivated commercially since the seventeenth century. Small, young white mushrooms are sold as button or crimini mushrooms, and those that are slightly larger and more mature are called closed-cap mushrooms. They have a white cap and almost no stem and their tender flesh can be eaten both raw and cooked. Closed-cap mushrooms have similar ivory-white caps but have developed gills. The flavour then deepens as the mushroom matures.

SERVING SUGGESTIONS
Cook in a Thai vegetable curry; stir-fry with oyster mushrooms, ginger or galangal, garlic and chilli; halve and sauté in oil and garlic; finely dice and add to salads; cook in vinegar and water with tarragon and lemon, or garlic and black pepper, or bay leaves, then leave to pickle before straining.

CHESTNUT MUSHROOMS

This bosky, brown-capped form of the common cultivated white mushroom is also known as the crimini mushroom or baby portobello. It has a meatier texture than button mushrooms and a more obvious 'mushroomy' flavour. Portobello is a chestnut mushroom that has matured for longer and has – for a cultivated mushroom – a particularly rich flavour.

SERVING SUGGESTIONS
Cook diced chestnut mushrooms in oil, then add finely chopped vacuum-packed cooked chestnuts and vegan cream and sage or parsley to make a sauce for

pasta; make mushroom and lentil burgers; combine chestnut mushrooms with a few rehydrated or fresh wild mushrooms to make a mushroom soup; sauté then use as a pizza topping; stir-fry with asparagus and shiitake mushrooms; roast portobello mushrooms whole, with a crispy breadcrumb and herb topping; make a mushroom paté or a bolognese-style sauce with finely chopped chestnut mushrooms; thinly slice and stir-fry, then add to noodles with a nut-based spicy sauce.

FLAT WHITE MUSHROOMS

These are full-grown button mushrooms with an almost flat, open cap. They have a more complex flavour than small white mushrooms.

SERVING SUGGESTIONS

Sauté in oil then stir in chopped tarragon; roast with butternut squash and serve with quinoa or bulgur wheat; sauté chopped mushrooms and onion with garlic to make a vegan duxelles then use as a filling for puff-pastry pies; slice thickly and fry with spices to use as a taco filling; slice, then fry with oil and herbs and serve on soft, warm polenta.

NUTRITIONAL BENEFITS OF MUSHROOMS

Rich in calcium, iron, magnesium, potassium, vitamin B_3, vitamin B_5, folic acid and zinc. In reaction to UV light, they naturally produce vitamin D: in order to activate this process, place mushrooms on a windowsill, gill side up, for an hour or two before using.

Dried mushrooms

In most cases, drying a mushroom intensifies its flavour, as the loss of water causes them to shrink. Morels, trompette, shiitake, oyster mushrooms and chanterelles can all be bought in dried form. Soak in warm water until rehydrated (soak oyster mushrooms for less time than brown varieties), and if you want to use the soaking water in a dish, soup or stock, strain it first to get rid of any grit or sand. Use a small amount of dried, rehydrated mushroom to enhance and deepen the flavour of a regular (blander) white or brown mushroom dish. Grind dried mushrooms to use as a seasoning, or buy them ready-ground.

TO DRY YOUR OWN MUSHROOMS:

- Slice fresh unblemished mushrooms, place in a single layer on a paper-lined tray and dry in the sun or in a warm, dry place for 2–3 days.
- Remove any dirt or debris with a brush, then store in a clean, airtight container.

Important:

Wash all wild mushrooms before using, and scrape the stem with a knife if necessary.

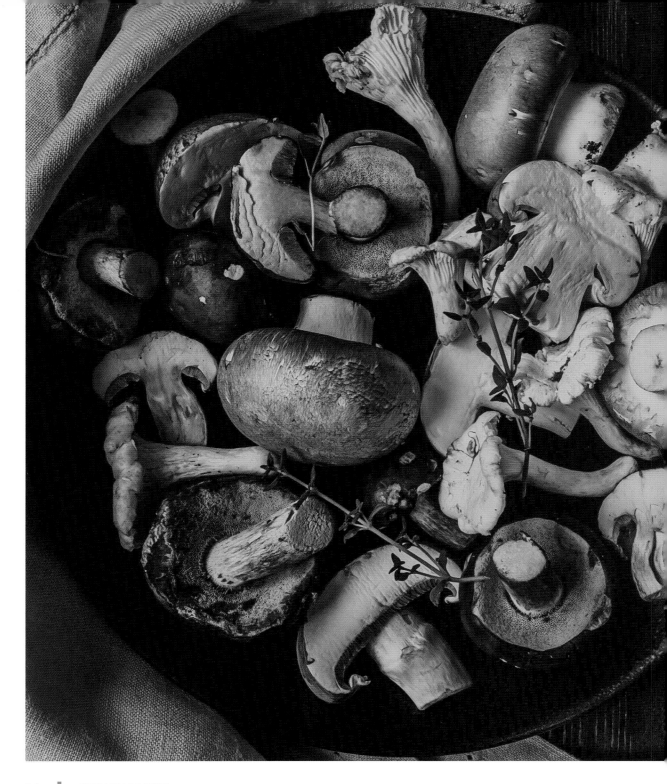

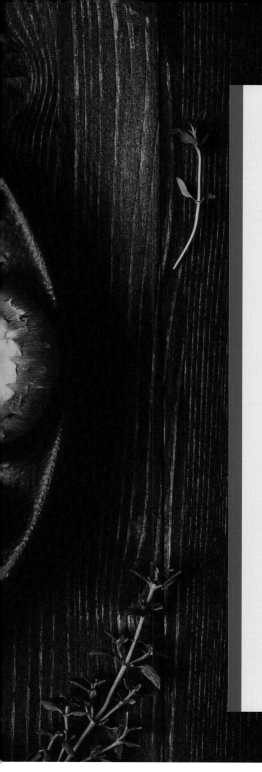

Other cultivated & wild mushroom varieties

OYSTER: A cultivated mushroom with fan-shaped cap, firm yet tender flesh and subtle flavour. The Japanese version is called hiratake or shimeji. The colour of the cap and stem varies with age, from bluish-grey to pale brown. Use in stir-fries and soups.

SHIITAKE: Make up around 25 per cent of the world's cultivated mushrooms and are widely used in Japanese and Chinese cuisine, where they are a key umami seasoning. They have a tan-coloured cap, white gills, a powerful flavour and firm meaty texture, and are best eaten when young. Remove stems before cooking, as they can be tough (use them in stock). Deep-fry, stir-fry or use in a miso-based or hot-and-sour soup.

FIELD: Field mushrooms are a wild species of mushroom with a white cap and thick white flesh, similar to the cultivated flat mushroom, and have similar culinary uses.

CHANTERELLE: This highly prized and expensive mushroom has a deep yolk colour, with a concave, funnel-shaped cap and fluted edge. Its colour signifies the presence of carotene, a source of vitamin A. The firm flesh has a nutty, fruity flavour and it remains firm when cooked. Grey chanterelles are known as girolles. Cook them gently: they are best suited to sautéing or a slow braise.

TROMPETTE: Also known as Horn of Plenty. A striking funnel-shaped mushroom with a fluted edge and deep gills. It ranges from dark brown to black in colour and has an intense and earthy flavour. Cut in half and brush out any dirt and debris before using.

MOREL: This mushroom is gathered in spring, rather than autumn, and is a highly prized delicacy. It has a conical cap with deep ridges that give it a crinkly honeycomb appearance, and its flavour is intense, smoky and meaty. Do not eat raw, and be sure to rinse and dry well before cooking. It requires a longer cooking time than most mushrooms.

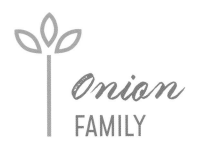

Onion FAMILY

Onions, garlic and leek are known as alliums and they all – in varying degrees – share the plant family's characteristic pungent scent and flavour. Native to northern temperate regions, the diverse variety of bulbs grow underground and range from mild, gently sweet and delicate in taste to piercingly sharp, tangy and earthy. They are rich in vitamins and minerals, can be eaten both raw and cooked and are vital ingredients in countless cuisines. The volatile compounds that give them their astringency break down during cooking and result in a milder taste and umami appeal. If you are eating them raw, rinse alliums in cold water first to temper their harsh sulphurous bite and feisty aroma. For chives, see page 135.

SPRING ONIONS

Spring onions (also known as salad onions or green onions) are tender, immature onions that are harvested while the leaves are still bright green. They have a milder, sweeter flavour than mature onion bulbs and the whole plant can be eaten, leaves and all. Some spring onions have a bulbous base, others are long and straight (like a baby leek). Calçots from Spain resemble young leeks and are traditionally served chargrilled, with a romesco sauce. Spring onions are used widely in Chinese cooking, often paired with ginger. To prolong their freshness, store them upright in the fridge, in a glass with some water in the bottom. In general, the thinner the spring onion, the milder it will be.

NUTRITIONAL BENEFITS
Similar to common onion.

SERVING SUGGESTIONS
Use finely chopped spring onion greens as a substitute for chives or in stir-fries; stir sliced spring onions through mashed potatoes; braise slowly with lettuce and peas; add chopped spring onions (green or white part, or both) to a tabbouleh; wilt spring onion tops in oil then scatter with roasted hazelnuts; serve whole and charred, with romesco sauce, a Catalan blend of garlic, nuts, tomatoes and chillies (sometimes also made with roasted red pepper); fry chopped spring onions with garlic and ginger as a base for a stir-fry.

SHALLOTS

This sub-species of onion, which grows in clusters of small bulbs, probably originated in central and southwestern Asia. It is popular in French cuisine, where it forms the foundation of many classic dishes, and in Asia they are fried until crisp and served over salads and broths (even desserts, on occasion). They can be eaten raw or cooked, and are often pickled (pickling varieties are sometimes called pearl onions or button onions). Shallots, and their elongated relative, banana shallots (also called echalion shallots), have a delicate and mild onion flavour. They don't take as well to browning as onions do, having a tendency to become bitter, so cook them slowly and gently or eat them raw.

NUTRITIONAL BENEFITS
Similar to common onion.

SERVING SUGGESTIONS
Sauté very slowly in oil until sweet and soft, for a vegan pissaladiére or puff pastry tart; caramelize in a frying pan with oil, rosemary or thyme, a little sugar and some red wine; pickle them whole; use in a *sambar* (Indian vegetable and lentil stew); finely chop, stir into a dressing and drizzle over freshly boiled new potatoes; thinly slice and fry in neutral oil until golden brown, to make crispy fried shallots, a perfect garnish for salads, dips, soups and other savoury dishes.

ONIONS

Countless meals begin with the chopping of an onion. This edible bulb has been cultivated and eaten for many thousands of years and is thought to have originated in central or western Asia. Today, it grows throughout temperate regions. It is a cornerstone vegetable in cuisines the world over and ranges widely in colour, from white, yellow and brown to purple and red. Some onions are mild and sweet, others can be highly pungent, with a harsh sulphurous 'sting' – in general, the younger and greener the onion, the more pungent it will be. Large Spanish onions (also known as yellow onions) and red onions are milder than large brown onions, so they are both good choices for eating raw. Diced with carrot and celery, onion makes a *mirepoix* or *soffritto*, a base used for all manner of savoury French and Italian dishes – in Cajun cooking the carrot is replaced by green pepper. They should be firm when pressed, and kept in a cool, dark place they store well.

NUTRITIONAL BENEFITS
A good source of calcium, magnesium, phosphorus, potassium, beta-carotene, folic acid and quercetin, vitamins A, C and E.

SERVING SUGGESTIONS
Soak sliced red onion in equal parts of sugar and wine vinegar for about an hour, then stir through cooked lentils or bulgur wheat (drained first, or include the sugar and vinegar) and sprinkle with sumac; roast onion wedges with oil and herbs, adding diced root vegetables if you like; make a deeply savoury-sweet onion soup, with just one type of onion, or a mixture of as many as you wish; make boulangére potatoes – a non-dairy version of a classic potato gratin – with sautéed onions, sliced potatoes, garlic, thyme and vegetable stock; slice and cook very slowly in oil then use as a filling for a savoury tart; make onion bhaji or fried onion rings; add pickled red onion rings to a tomato salad; boil unpeeled, whole onions for about 20 minutes, then drain, drizzle with oil, sprinkle with herbs, season and bake in foil until soft and golden.

tip

Add a little brown onion skin to stocks, broths and soups to add a golden colour, removing it before serving.

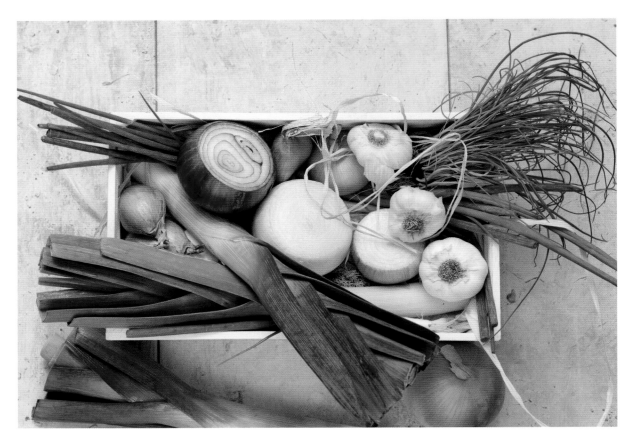

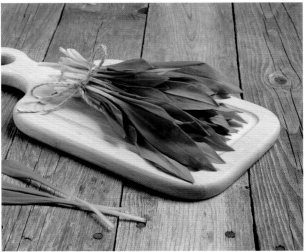

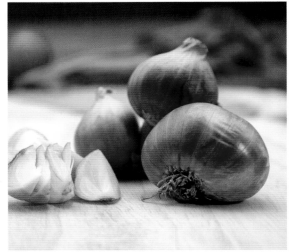

LEEKS

Cultivated by the ancient Egyptians and thought of highly by the Greeks and Romans, leeks have a mild, delicate flavour and a straight, elongated cylindrical bulb. The green tops are less tender than the white parts but contain more nutrients and have a deeper flavour. Wash before using, as soil and grit often gets trapped within the layers: make a long slit lengthways down the leek, just to the middle, then hold them under cold running water and rinse between each layer (or slice widthways into rounds and soak in cold water). Avoid letting them brown when cooking, as this causes them to become bitter and lose their sweet taste. Baby leeks can be eaten raw once thinly sliced.

NUTRITIONAL BENEFITS

A good source of potassium, vitamin K, calcium, folic acid, vitamins C, B_6 and A.

SERVING SUGGESTIONS

Use the green tops in stocks, soups and stews; braise sliced leeks with wine and herbs; make leek and potato soup; poach leeks whole, then grill them on a barbecue, letting the outer leaves blacken before peeling and serving the tender inner layers with a piquant dip; finely shred and fry green leek tops to use as a garnish for soups and salads; steam baby leeks, leave to cool and serve whole with vinaigrette.

Wild garlic

You can sniff out wild garlic in woodland long before you see it. It grows in spring and is a foragers' and farmers' market favourite. The pungent glossy green leaves, rich in vitamin C and beta-carotene, pack a garlicky punch and should be used as soon as possible after picking. Add chopped leaves to savoury scones, pesto, a fresh green herb sauce and bread doughs, or cook them with wild mushrooms. The star-shaped white flowers that emerge at the end of the wild garlic season are edible: sprinkle them on salads.

GARLIC

Long celebrated for its medicinal virtues and notorious for its pungency, garlic is thought to have evolved from the wild garlic of Central Asia and has been widely used for millennia. It is available fresh, dried or powdered and used as both a flavouring and a vegetable in its own right. There are two types: soft-neck and hard-neck. The soft-neck, creamy-white 'wet' (new season) garlic has a milder, subtle astringency. As it develops, the bulb swells and forms separate cloves within a white, pinkish or purple skin, which dries to form the familiar mature garlic, which is the most powerfully flavoured member of the allium family. Garlic is used to enhance the flavours of ingredients its paired with, but also works well as a key ingredient. The more you crush raw garlic, the stronger its pungency. On cooking (as long as it is not browned or burnt), the volatile sulphur compounds are transformed into savoury and mellow sweetness, even nuttiness. Elephant garlic is milder than garlic and is actually part of the leek family.

NUTRITIONAL BENEFITS

A rich source of potassium and other minerals, vitamins B_1 and C.

SERVING SUGGESTIONS

To add a mild garlic flavour to a cooked dish, add a whole clove to oil, heat gently, then remove the clove and use the oil; add raw chopped garlic to marinades for barbecued vegetables and to fresh salsas; bake young garlic with new potatoes; add young garlic cloves to the base for a risotto; roast mature bulbs whole in foil then add the sweet garlic pulp to a cauliflower, carrot or broad bean purée, dips or salad dressings; rub a cut garlic clove over toast; add to a Mexican mole sauce; blitz young garlic with fresh herbs and oil to make pesto; make a gremolata with lemon, parsley and garlic; make the cold Spanish soup, *ajo blanco*, with blanched almonds, stale bread, garlic, sherry vinegar, oil, ice-cold water and cucumber; blitz garlic and ginger to a paste and use as a base for curries and marinades.

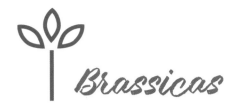

Brassicas

Brassicas are believed to have evolved over thousands of years from a wild kale-like cabbage native to European coastal regions, and have developed to form a vast array of leafy vegetables.

Cabbages have been cultivated for millennia, with many species bred to form the tight, round cabbage heads we're familiar with today. Their many virtues have often been overshadowed by a reputation for filling kitchens with a nasty smell, due to the sulphurous compounds released when the vegetable is overcooked, but with judicious preparation they offer subtle succulence, freshness and a host of valuable nutrients. The waxy, succulent leaves can be eaten raw or cooked: raw, they share a fresh 'bite' similar to that of mustard and a grassy aroma, and when cooked their sweetness is enhanced. Cabbages should feel heavy and solid, with no discolouration.

Broccoli and cauliflower are thought to have been bred from flowering cabbage shoots to form branching, compact clusters of tiny buds (undeveloped flowers), but which came first – the broccoli or cauliflower – is not certain. Brassicas, particularly the stems of broccoli and cauliflower, are rich in dietary fibre, vitamin C and beta-carotene.

SAVOY CABBAGES

This robustly-textured winter cabbage was developed in Europe in the Middle Ages. Fuller in flavour than white or red cabbage, it has wrinkly green leaves that form a loose head and have a satisfying crunch. The thicker outer leaves are used in many cuisines to encase and bake savoury fillings. Trim away the tough core before using the leaves. Soaking the cut leaves in cold water for a short time before cooking helps get rid of any bitterness. Green outer leaves contain more carotene than paler inner leaves.

NUTRITIONAL BENEFITS
Rich in beta-carotene, iron and vitamin K, and a good source of vitamin C.

SERVING SUGGESTIONS
Shred and sauté in a pan with oil and caraway seeds (and garlic, if you wish) until just tender; shred and stir-fry briefly in Indian-spiced oil (coriander, cumin, curry leaves, mustard seeds, turmeric); blanch or steam whole leaves, drain, then stuff with a mixture of cooked rice or lentils, onion, chopped nuts and herbs, before baking with tomato sauce; make a ribollita by sautéing onions, carrots, celery, leek, adding tomatoes, cannellini beans and vegetable stock and simmering, then stir through shredded cabbage when it's almost ready to serve; serve raw in salads, with a citrusy dressing.

RED CABBAGES

Red cabbage has a sweeter, earthier flavour than white, though the dark magenta leaves take longer to cook. It is eaten both raw and cooked. The nutrient-dense leaves will turn purply-blue when heated, unless an acid such as fruit, wine or vinegar is added in the cooking process. Red cabbage contains a plant chemical called anthocyanin which has been shown to help reduce the risk of heart disease. It keeps well.

NUTRITIONAL BENEFITS
Rich in vitamin C and vitamin A. Contains more vitamin K, iron and vitamin A than white cabbage.

SERVING SUGGESTIONS
Braise red cabbage slowly with apple, onion, juniper berries or star anise, bay, sugar and vinegar; make a coleslaw with carrot, onion, fennel, mustard, vegan yoghurt or tahini dressing, and fresh herbs; shred and stir into a noodle soup just before serving; shred and combine with grated carrot, beetroot and chopped dates; stir-fry with chopped chestnuts.

WHITE CABBAGES

Also known as Dutch cabbage, white cabbage is a firm, pale variety of round-headed cabbage, with tightly packed leaves. It is often eaten raw in salads or preserved in a pickle or ferment, and sauerkraut and cabbage soup have played a crucial role in Russian culinary culture over the past three centuries. It keeps well.

NUTRITIONAL BENEFITS
A good source of vitamin K, vitamin C, magnesium and folate.

SERVING SUGGESTIONS
Shred and add to an Asian-style coleslaw tossed with a peanut and chilli dressing; make sauerkraut – fermented cabbage – by mixing thinly sliced cabbage in a bowl with fine sea salt (or rock salt) and caraway seeds, leave it to stand for about 20 minutes, then pack into a sterilized

container, including any juices from the bowl; to make a quick pickle, finely shred cabbage, add vinegar, honey, coriander or fennel seeds, ginger and chilli and combine (use within an hour or two); shred and add to Vietnamese summer rolls with beansprouts and other shredded vegetables, and serve with a peanut and soy dipping sauce; cut into thick wedges, drizzle with oil and roast until tender.

BRUSSELS SPROUTS

Brussels sprouts come from a cabbage variant that was developed in Europe less than 500 years ago to produce small, compact heads on an elongated stalk. Synonymous with the Christmas feast, this miniature sub-species of cabbage has an appealing nuttiness, yet also and a strong bitterness which can be off-putting to some. This bitterness can be minimized by halving and blanching them briefly in boiling water before roasting or pan-frying. If you grow or buy sprouts intact on their stalk, with the sprout tops, cook the tops as you would spring greens (see page 74). They are best in winter months and can be eaten raw or cooked.

NUTRITIONAL BENEFITS
Rich in calcium, magnesium, iron, phosphorus, potassium, beta-carotene, B vitamins, vitamin C, K and E, and folic acid.

SERVING SUGGESTIONS
Pan-fry shredded sprouts in oil with a pinch of chilli flakes and some garlic and ginger, or with chopped cooked chestnuts; chop and add to a stir-fry or fried rice; slice thinly, sauté and stir through mashed potato to make bubble and squeak; steam briefly and sprinkle with grated nutmeg before serving.

BROCCOLI

Native to the eastern Mediterranean, broccoli was not widely known in Europe until the seventeenth or eighteenth century. A member of the cabbage family, it is characterized by tiny (typically green) buds that form in clusters and are recognized in three forms: calabrese – one head with a fleshy stalk, sprouting broccoli – smaller, separate flower heads (purple, green or white) on long, individual stalks, and romanesco – yellowish-green groups of multiple heads clustered together that resemble a cauliflower head. Calabrese is succulent and mild, and sprouting broccoli tends to have a more full-bodied, earthy, iron flavour. Romanesco has a nutty, slightly sweet flavour that sits somewhere between broccoli and cauliflower, and photogenic clusters of buds in tight, fractal cones. All three forms of broccoli should be cooked only briefly. Adding a little mustard to cooked broccoli boosts its ability to generate a protective compound called sulphoraphane (the same applies to cabbage, Brussels sprouts and kale).

NUTRITIONAL BENEFITS
Contains large amounts of minerals, vitamin A, folic acid and calcium, and more vitamin C than oranges.

SERVING SUGGESTIONS
Trim broccoli stems with a vegetable peeler and eat raw or chop and add to a stir-fry, soup or sauté in oil; blanch florets and stem in salted boiling water, toss in a pan with sautéed onions and garlic, then serve with pasta and a sprinkle of toasted breadcrumbs and fresh herbs and capers; steam to retain the most nutrients; add florets to a Chinese stir-fry with tofu and ginger; roast florets in olive oil, then dress with lemon and sprinkle with toasted pine nuts; if cooking whole, boil broccoli or sprouting broccoli standing up in the pan if possible, so the heads do not overcook; roast romanesco florets with cherry tomatoes then toss through a lentil salad.

CAULIFLOWERS

A mild-mannered member of the cabbage family. Cauliflower is thought to have originated in the eastern Mediterranean before becoming popular in Europe in the 1500s. The creamy-white head has densely-packed curds (florets) and both the curds and the short central stem have a delicate, earthy flavour which, develops a musky nuttiness and satisfying savoury depth when cooked. If overcooked, its sulphurous flavour can be unpleasant. The edible leaves are tender and sweet. The more you cut it, the more sulphurous it tastes. Purple and orange varieties contain more phytochemicals than the white variety.

NUTRITIONAL BENEFITS
A rich source of potassium, iron and zinc, and contains vitamins A and C.

SERVING SUGGESTIONS
Blanch florets, then pickle in sweetened and/or spiced wine vinegar; add small raw florets to salads; roast whole heads brushed with spiced oil, along with the green leaves; add the leaves and florets to a stir-fry; make a cauliflower and chickpea curry; make a purée by adding florets to sautéed onion, adding non-dairy milk, simmering until tender, then blitzing until smooth (roast the cauliflower first if you prefer a deeper flavour); deep-fry florets dredged in a tempura or spiced chickpea flour batter, then serve with a chilli or tamari dipping sauce; make aloo gobi; roast florets with cumin, cinnamon and ginger, then toss through a lentil, preserved lemon and leafy-green salad topped with toasted almonds; grate or blitz to make cauliflower rice; chargrill thick slices, then serve with a tahini dressing.

tip

Broccoli's taste softens on cooking, whereas cauliflower's flavour deepens and becomes more mustardy.

Other cabbage varieties

KOHLRABI: a thick-skinned, swollen stem in the cabbage family with a crisp texture and mild flavour similar to broccoli stalk. It resembles a turnip and can be eaten raw or cooked briefly as you might a parsnip or celeriac.

SWEDE: this peppery-sweet, starchy swollen stem is a cross between the turnip and cabbage species. It can be white or yellow and is often boiled and mashed but can also be eaten raw.

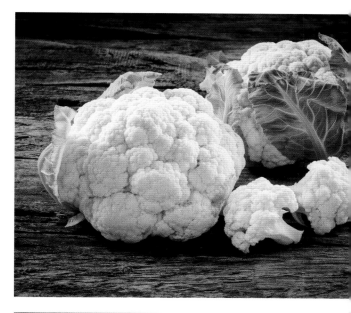

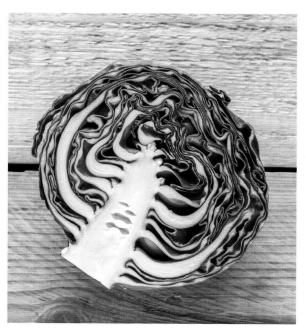

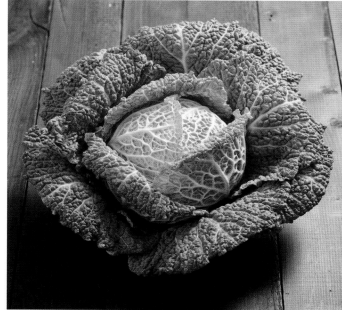

Leafy greens

Arguably the most versatile of all vegetables, leafy greens can be incorporated into almost any meal and have been a winter staple for millennia. Rich in fibre, these open-leaved plants accumulate more vitamins C and A and carotenoids than ones with leaves that are closely nested around the tip of the main plant stalk (such as cabbage). Fresh young leaves are the least fibrous and have the most delicate flavour. The darker the leaf, the richer it is in vitamins and minerals.

KALE

Descended from the wild cabbages of Europe, kale was a common green vegetable in Europe until the Middle Ages, when round-headed cabbages started making an appearance. The hardy winter greens have a robust, earthy flavour and meaty texture. Curly kale, the most widely available variety, has tough ribs that should be removed before cooking, unless the leaves are very young (if the rib snaps cleanly, it should be tender enough to cook and eat). Tuscan cavolo nero has long, very dark green (almost blue-black) crinkled leaves. Red Russian kale has a purple tinge and small frilly leaves: the leaves are softer than regular kale and only require brief cooking.

NUTRITIONAL BENEFITS
A rich source of magnesium, vitamins A and C, calcium and B vitamins.

SERVING SUGGESTIONS
Blanch in boiling salted water, then drain, squeeze out excess liquid and sauté in olive oil with sliced garlic; make the hearty Tuscan soup ribollita with cavolo nero, cannellini beans, bread, onion, celery, garlic and tomatoes; massage the trimmed leaves in a bowl with oil thoroughly for a few minutes, to tenderize, then spread out on a baking sheet, season with spices, salt and/or nutritional yeast and bake in the oven until crisp (massaging them with oil tenderizes them sufficiently to be eaten raw in a salad, too); juice with apples or carrot.

SPRING GREENS

This hardy loose-leaf cabbage, a member of the brassica family, has a loose head of green leaves with paler yellow-green inner leaves in the centre. The leaves have a tender, silky texture and sweet, subtle cabbage taste once cooked. Although their name suggests otherwise, spring greens are available all year round. The darker leaves require a longer cooking time and are more strongly flavoured than the lighter inner leaves. 'Spring greens' is also used as a term to describe the young leafy greens of other brassicas such as cauliflower, broccoli, turnip and kale.

NUTRITIONAL BENEFITS
A good source of vitamins C, E and K, iron, potassium, fibre and calcium.

SERVING SUGGESTIONS
Steam and stir-fry the leaves with chilli and garlic, then add a squeeze of lemon juice and serve scattered with toasted hazelnuts; roll up the leaves and shred them finely, then deep-fry in oil until crisp to make 'crispy

seaweed'; slice into ribbons and stir into a coconut dhal or chickpea and squash curry; shred, blanch and stir through a cannellini bean stew; steam sliced spring greens and stir through a warm quinoa or bulgur wheat salad with a tahini or citrusy mustard dressing; braise with wild garlic.

CHARD

Although it resembles spinach and has a similar earthy flavour, chard is in fact a variety of beetroot that has been bred to produce broad, meaty leaf stalks. Both the large, crinkly, dark green leaves and the stalks have a stronger minerally sweet flavour and slightly coarser texture than spinach. The colour of the stalks of rainbow chard varieties varies from white to bright red, purple and yellow (the red-stalked varieties have a beetroot-like sweetness). Swiss chard, a hardier variety than the coloured-stalk chard, has white stems and particularly fleshy stalks. Young chard leaves can be eaten raw, but mature, larger leaves benefit from a brief blanch or sauté. Separate the leaves and stalks of large chard and cook the stalks for longer.

NUTRITIONAL BENEFITS
Rich in vitamins K, C and A, magnesium, iron and potassium.

SERVING SUGGESTIONS
Use the stalks and leaves in a French savoury tian made with courgette, garlic, onion, cooked rice and vegan cheese; make *marak silk*, a Moroccan tagine, with chard leaves and stalks slowly sautéed with onion, coriander and paprika, before adding rice and a little water and cooking until the rice is cooked; stir into a hot vegetable stew or risotto; sauté with garlic, oil and lemon; use small leaves raw in salads.

SPINACH

Believed to have been first cultivated in Persia during the fourth century AD, spinach was introduced to Europe in the late Middle Ages, and widespread cultivation began in the eighteenth century. Spinach is used as both a salad green and vegetable: the young, mild and tender leaves can be eaten raw and its subtle, bitter-sweet earthy taste works well in myriad cooked dishes. The acidic tang it has in its raw state disappears when heated. It cooks down significantly, to about a tenth of its original volume, as the leaves are mostly composed of water. Trim away large, tough stalks on mature leaves before cooking.

NUTRITIONAL BENEFITS
Rich in vitamin A and folic acid, beta-carotene, potassium, iron, vitamin B_6, calcium, vitamin E and magnesium. An excellent source of vitamin C, if eaten raw.

SERVING SUGGESTIONS
Add wilted, chopped spinach to gnocchi dough; stir through an Indian vegetable curry; rinse spinach leaves thoroughly, drain, then put in a frying pan with the water still clinging to them, cover and cook until wilted before draining again – drizzle with oil and grate over fresh nutmeg and some finely grated lemon zest; serve fresh leaves topped with fried tofu 'croutons'; make the Greek spinach pie, spanakopita, using tofu instead of feta; blitz with toasted pine nuts, basil and oil to make pesto.

Chinese and Asian leafy greens

Most Chinese and Asian greens are members of the brassica family (cabbage and mustard plants) and can be eaten in similar ways, typically cooked over a high heat for a short amount time. They range in flavour from peppery hot to sweet and mild and most have tender leaves.

PAK CHOI: Also known as Chinese celery cabbage and Chinese white cabbage, pak choi has pale fleshy stalks and smooth, glossy green leaves with a mild mustardy flavour that tastes like a cross between white cabbage and spinach. It is more closely related to turnips than cabbages. Baby pak choi can be cooked whole.

CHINESE SPINACH: Also known as *yin choi*, Chinese spinach is not botanically related to spinach, but its leaves have a similar taste. Small, young leaves can be eaten raw.

CHINESE LEAVES: Also known as Napa cabbage, this vegetable resembles a very large head of celery. The pale green, crinkly leaves have long, broad white ribs and have a crunchy texture and mild cabbage flavour but none of the associated sulphurous flavour. They can be eaten fresh or cooked and are typically used in salads, soups, stews and stir-fries.

CHINESE MUSTARD GREENS: Also known as *gai choi*. The deep green leaves are quite fiery. Like spinach, the young leaves can be eaten raw, but older, more strongly-flavoured leaves are better stir-fried or blanched.

CHOI SUM: Also known as Chinese flowering cabbage and *yu choi*, this vegetable is related to oilseed rape. It has bright yellow flowers, green leaves and thin pale green stalks and is usually sold in bunches. The delicately flavoured leaves are often steamed.

CHINESE BROCCOLI: Also called Chinese kale, Chinese broccoli has a stronger flavour than *choi sum* and white flowers rather than yellow. It comes from the same family as mustard greens and the long slender stems and loose leaves have a robust taste and coarser texture. Every part of the plant is eaten (often stir-fried) and the peeled stems are considered a delicacy.

WATER SPINACH: also known as *tong choi*, water spinach has hollow stalks, narrow pointed leaves and a similar flavour to spinach.

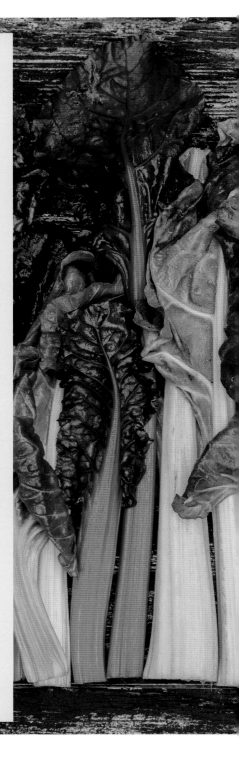

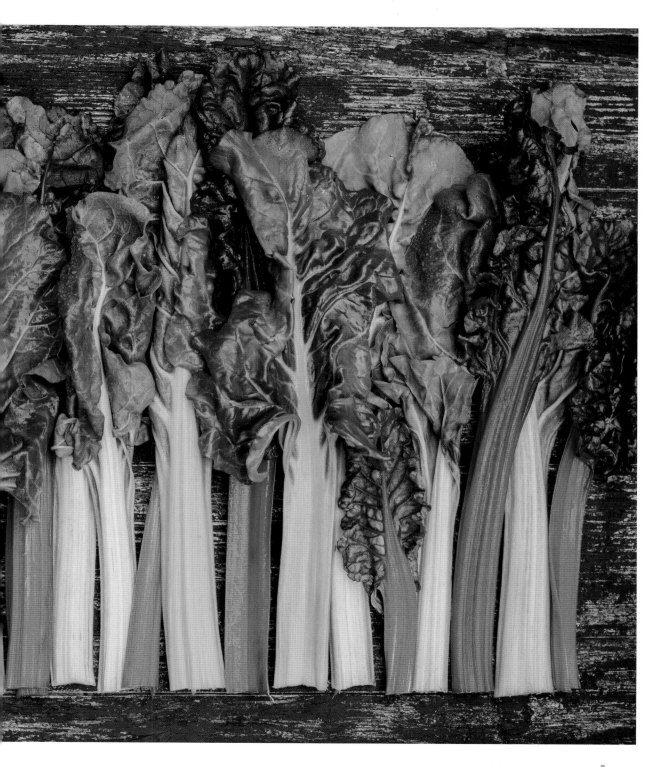

Salad leaves

CHICORY AND ENDIVE: Used as a vegetable and a salad leaf since classical times. They have been bred over time to become less bitter, though they still have a pleasing bite. Both chicory and endive have firm, crunchy and refreshing leaves that are nutritionally similar to lettuce (endive is particularly rich in folic acid). Chicory – also, confusingly, known as Belgian endive – has pale spear-shaped leaves and true endive, a close relation of chicory, is slightly less bitter and available in two types: curly-leaf (frisée) and broadleaf (batavia/escarole). Broadleaf endive is less bitter than curly. Serving chicory or endive with fatty or sweet ingredients, or blanching them, mellows their bitterness. They are eaten fresh and often braised and grilled.

RADICCHIO: This red-leaf chicory is popular in Italy. There are three key types: round-headed radicchio, which has a bitter-sweet flavour and is best used in salads; Treviso, which has pointed leaves on a long, tapered head and is largely used for cooking; and Castelfranco, a loose-headed chicory with light green leaves streaked with red. The firm-textured leaves are often wilted and used as a ravioli stuffing in Italy, served in salads or grilled.

MUSTARD AND CRESS: These young plants are sold, often together, as sprouted seedlings for use in salads ('cress' sold commercially in punnets is often salad rape). Cress is feathery and mild and mustard cress is darker green and fiery, with small, heart-shaped leaves. They are rich in carotenes and vitamin C.

ROCKET: Strong and peppery, rocket is native to the Mediterranean and has been used as a salad plant since classical times. Younger leaves have a milder taste and the leaves are more tender. Make rocket pesto by combining it with a more mildly-flavoured leaf such as spinach.

LETTUCE: Lettuce has been cultivated since antiquity, though the lettuces then were loose and headless types – round and firm-headed lettuces didn't appear until around the sixteenth century. They are the most popular leafy salad vegetable, with colours ranging from green to red to spotted. Lettuce is a good source of beta-carotene, magnesium, potassium and folic acid, as well as vitamins C and E, particularly in green-leaf varieties.

Butterhead: Pliable, rounded leaves form a soft head of lettuce. The leaves are tender and have an agreeably mild, sweet flavour.

Cos/romaine: Long-leaf lettuce. It has the crispness of iceberg and the advantage of a full-bodied 'green' taste. Red-freckled varieties have a buttery texture and sweet taste.

Iceberg: Crisp, tightly compacted, firm lettuce. The pale green leaves have little flavour – it's the crisp texture that gives it appeal in salads and sandwiches.

Little Gem: Sweet, small variety of cos lettuce. Popular cooked and raw (try it braised quartered or halved in vegetable stock with mint and peas).

Lamb's lettuce: Also known as corn salad and mâche. The small, dark green leaves have a subtle flavour and are eaten fresh, not cooked.

WATERCRESS: This member of the mustard family has a biting, pungent taste and mineral freshness. The dark green leaves and stems are rich in calcium, magnesium, phosphorus, potassium, vitamins C and A, and beta-carotene. It's usually eaten raw as a salad or garnish, or in soup.

RADISHES

This crunchy, peppery taproot from the cabbage family is thought to be native to western Asia. It was cultivated in ancient Rome and Greece and reached Britain by the sixteenth century, heading to the New World not long after. Varieties range widely in size, shape and colour and fall into three types: western/small, winter and oriental. All have different levels of pepperiness, though the texture and flavour profile is similar and most have smooth, edible skins. Of the western varieties, the elongated French Breakfast and round, scarlet Cherry radish are the most widely known (French Breakfast has a milder – some say more delicate – flavour than most). Daikon ('mooli' in India and the West Indies), a popular radish in Japan and Korea, is white and long and has mild, juicy flesh – it is typically thinly sliced or pickled. Black winter radish features in Eastern European cuisines and has robust, pungent flesh that is often grated or pickled.

All radishes should be firm and the freshest taste the sweetest. Buy with the edible leafy tops attached, if possible. Put them in a bowl of iced water to refresh them before serving. Cooking radishes tames their peppery heat.

NUTRITIONAL BENEFITS
A good source of calcium, magnesium, potassium, phosphorus, beta-carotene, folic acid and vitamin C. Daikon contains twice as much vitamin C as red radishes but less iron and calcium.

SERVING SUGGESTIONS
Thinly slice and add to salads with a citrusy dressing (oranges complement radish well) and fresh herbs; make a radish salsa with shallots and coriander; ferment with spices to make Korean kimchi; pickle sliced radishes in a solution of salt, sugar, white wine vinegar, lemon and dill; halve French Breakfast radishes and sauté them in oil with tarragon or thyme, add a little stock or wine; stir-fry with other greens; cook young piquant radish leaves as you would spinach (fresh or cooked); roast tossed in oil and rosemary (and maple syrup, if you like).

AVOCADOS

Native to Central America and Mexico and cultivated for over 7,000 years, avocados now grow in nearly all tropical and sub-tropical regions. The oil-rich fruit was considered a novelty in Europe until recent times. Each fruit is pear-shaped or round, contains creamy green-yellow flesh and a single large seed. More than twenty varieties are cultivated, but the most popular are recognized as two distinct types: the Californian 'Hass', which is small with brown-black, leathery and lumpy skin and the paler type grown in Florida (such as Fuerte and Ettinger), which are larger and smooth-skinned. Hass are largely considered to have a superior taste and tend to be richer in oil than smooth-skinned varieties.

Avocados are usually eaten fresh, though they can be briefly cooked. The buttery flesh has a mild nuttiness and grass-like taste, contains 15–30 per cent monounsaturated fat and is a good source of protein, carbohydrate, vitamins and minerals. It browns quickly once cut, however. To prevent discolouration, rub or sprinkle the flesh with lemon or lime juice. To test for ripeness, press gently at the stalk end: it should yield just a little. They can be bought hard and ripened at home (refrigerate only after they are fully ripened).

NUTRITIONAL BENEFITS
Rich in potassium (they contain about the same amount as bananas), iron, copper, phosphorus, beta-carotene, folic acid, vitamins A, B, K and E.

SERVING SUGGESTIONS
Mash ripe avocado with lime juice, chilli and coriander to make guacamole; add to a smoothie or raw pea and cucumber soup; cube and add to black bean burritos, tacos or quesadillas with tomato salsa; Latin American soup; smash avocado with tender broad beans, oil and lemon to serve on toast; pair with grilled peaches or nectarines (or mangoes), wild rice beans and roasted vegetables in a taco; blitz with herbs, lime juice and non-dairy yoghurt to make a creamy dressing; add to vegetable and rice sushi rolls or Vietnamese spring rolls; blitz with cocoa powder, lime juice and maple syrup to make a sweet mousse; blitz with herbs and toasted nuts to make a pesto.

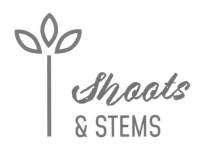

Shoots & STEMS

These plants are grown for their young stems and leaf stalks, to be eaten as vegetables or salad ingredients. Some are tender in nature, others only become tender when cooked.

ASPARAGUS

Asparagus is native to Central and southern Europe, North Africa and western and Central Asia. It was cultivated in ancient times and appreciated as a delicacy. It fell off the culinary map in the Middle Ages, however, before regaining popularity in the seventeenth century. The young shoots, known as 'spears', herald the arrival of spring produce and are harvested by hand during their short season. White asparagus is green asparagus that is covered in soil as it grows, to prevent exposure to sunlight and the production of chlorophyll. It is more fibrous than green or purple asparagus and has a milder flavour. Tender green and purple spears have an assertive sweet, nutty and sulphurous flavour and contain more nutrients than white. Asparagus quickly loses its sweetness, so eat as soon as possible after buying. The buds should be tight and the spears firm. Trim the woody base (use these in soup or stock). Cook upright if possible, so that the spears are in the water and the tips cook in the steam. Storing them upright in a container of shallow water in the fridge helps keep them fresh.

NUTRITIONAL BENEFITS
A rich source of vitamins C, E and K, iron, potassium and folic acid and beta-carotene.

SERVING SUGGESTIONS
Shave tender spears to eat raw in salads; make an asparagus risotto, adding the tough bases to the stock (but not the risotto) to boost the asparagus flavour; cook on a griddle or barbecue, then dress with olive oil and lemon juice, orange juice or vinegar; trim, slice and add to a stir-fry; serve warm with new potatoes; blanch, chop and add to a cold noodle and cucumber salad with a peanut or miso-based dressing; slice and sauté with shallots, peas and lemon zest, then serve with pasta, topped with fried breadcrumbs or toasted nuts; roast with diced celeriac, tofu, turnip, cauliflower florets or fennel.

FENNEL

There are three types of cultivated fennel: bitter fennel, sweet fennel (grown for use as a herb) and Florence/Italian fennel (the sweet type we eat as a vegetable). They all belong to the parsley family. Fennel has been appreciated as a vegetable and seed (spice – see page 150) since the classical era, possibly earlier, and was introduced to Britain in the seventeenth or early eighteenth century. The large bulbous leaf base of Florence fennel is composed of tightly overlapping stems that have a crisp texture and clean, anise taste with citrusy notes when eaten raw, which sweetens and mellows when cooked until soft. Store fennel trimmings in the freezer to add to the pan when you make a stock. If a fennel bulb comes with its feathery fronds intact, use them in salads or to garnish dishes – they have a milder anise flavour than the bulb.

NUTRITIONAL BENEFITS
A rich source of potassium, folic acid and minerals, fennel also carotenes, calcium, vitamins A, C, E, K and B.

Slice thinly and eat raw with a squeeze of lemon; add to a salad of watercress, rocket and orange; blanch, then char thick slices on a griddle or barbecue before dressing with olive oil and lemon; sauté chopped fennel with onion to make the base for a risotto; braise slowly with onions and use to top flatbread or pizza; add thinly sliced fennel to a green cabbage sauerkraut; roast with diced celeriac; blanch, then coat in batter and deep-fry; braise halved bulbs in a little white wine with olive oil and lemon juice; simmer until tender, then drain and purée with olive oil.

CELERY

Celery originates from a wild, hollow-stemmed bitter green plant in the parsley family (sometimes called 'smallage') that is native to temperate shorelines and marshes. It was popular in Roman times as a flavouring rather than a vegetable, until it was bred to grow a more tender, sweeter leaf stalk in the seventeenth and eighteenth centuries. Modern cultivated celery contains about 95 per cent water and has a subtle, slightly nutty anise flavour and a juicy, tangy crunch. Green and white celery are the same plant, grown differently: white/pale green celery is blanched (earth is piled up against the emerging plant), or comes from a self-blanching variety, and has a gentler taste than green, which is a little more astringent and peppery. It can be eaten raw or cooked. The inner stems are the most tender. If necessary, use a peeler to remove the stringy fibres from outer layers. Stalks should be firm and stiff. If celery comes with leaves, use them in salads or soups.

NUTRITIONAL BENEFITS
A good source of potassium and a negligible amount of minerals, some vitamin B$_3$, folic acid and beta-carotenes.

SERVING SUGGESTIONS
Braise celery hearts slowly in stock or water; roast celery with onions, herbs and olive oil, then blitz with stock to make a soup; add to stock; sauté with chopped onions and carrots to make a sweet base (also known as a mirepoix or soffrito) for a vegetable soup; slice the tender inner stalks and add to a bowl with walnuts and apple to make a salad (celery shares a similar flavour compound with walnuts); use celery leaves in salads and soups; stir-fry chopped celery with ginger.

GLOBE ARTICHOKES

Artichokes come from a thistle-like plant – a cousin of the cardoon native to Europe and North Africa that has been bred to produce various varieties of flower heads. The immature heads are made up of hard, tightly overlapping leaves (bracts) that have edible, succulent bases beneath hairy fibres (known as the choke), which are inedible. Artichokes were cultivated and valued as a vegetable in Greek and Roman times and have long been popular in Italian cuisine. They range from green to purple/violet and have a complex earthy, nutty-sweet flavour, buttery texture and sizes ranging from tiny buds to large heads. They are usually cooked, but miniature artichokes can be eaten whole (raw or cooked), as the hairy choke has not yet formed and the leaves haven't hardened. The tender hearts are often sold in tins. Miniature artichokes can be served raw. Artichokes have the unusual effect of making anything you eat straight after taste artificially sweet.

NUTRITIONAL BENEFITS
Rich in iron and minerals and a good source of vitamins B, C and K, calcium, magnesium, phosphorus, potassium, zinc and folic acid.

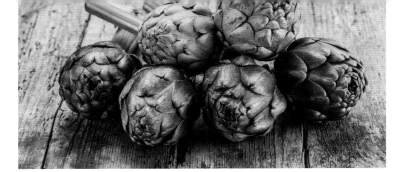

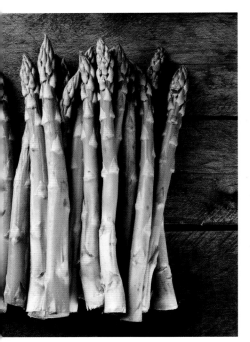

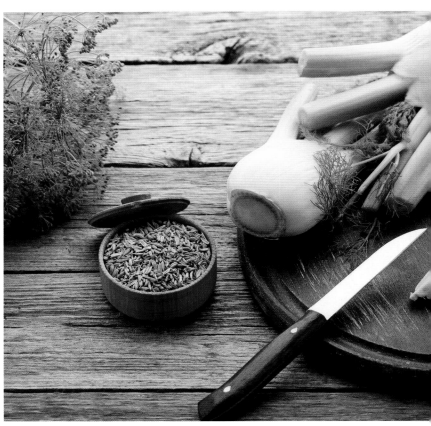

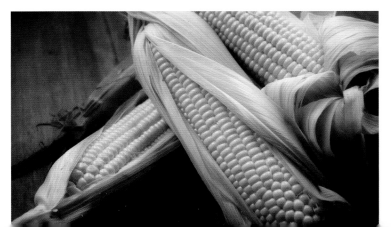

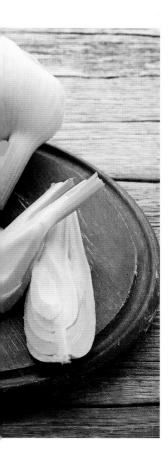

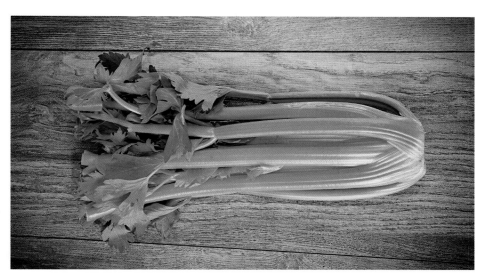

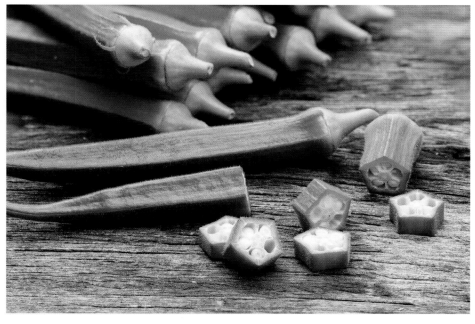

To prepare a large artichoke, remove the stem, prise open the leaves, scrape out the choke, then rinse. Boil in salted water with a little lemon juice until tender (10–30 minutes). Alternatively, remove the leaves and hairy choke before cooking, and just cook the hearts. To eat whole boiled artichokes (warm or cold), pull off the leaves, dip them into a sharp dressing and scrape off the tender base of each leaf with your teeth, until you reach the heart. Remove the choke before eating the heart. Boil small violet artichokes whole until tender, then trim away tough outer leaves, halve and remove the hairy choke. Use cooked artichoke heart in risottos, braise, or purée with tinned white beans and lemon juice to make a dip. Shave miniature artichokes into a salad or deep-fry whole.

OKRA

Also known as lady's fingers, okro and bhindi, this member of the mallow family grows in tropical and sub-tropical regions throughout the world and is harvested when immature. Okra has a mild, sweet vegetal flavour not unlike runner beans. Its thick, gummy juice (which divides opinion and is considered either virtuous or vile) helps thicken cooked dishes, particularly in West Africa, India, the Middle East, the Caribbean and the Americas: in Creole and Cajun food, it gives 'gumbo soups' their glutinous character. The firm, ridged seed pods are mostly green, but red are also sometimes available (some red varieties turn green when cooked, others retain their colour). If you want to reduce the stickiness, soak the pods in water with a little lemon juice before cooking and cook them whole – with stem trimmed off – rather than sliced. Their gelatinous qualities increase the longer they are cooked.

NUTRITIONAL BENEFITS
A good source of calcium, magnesium, zinc, B vitamins, phosphorus, potassium, vitamin C and omega-3 fatty acids.

SERVING SUGGESTIONS
Roast whole, drizzled with oil, for 30 minutes, or until tender; dip in batter, then deep-fry; add to a tomato-based vegetable curry along with green beans; roast briefly so the okra is still firm, then add to a dhal or coconut curry; halve lengthways and fry in a little oil until crisp; pickle in a sweet, vinegary brine with mustard seeds, peppercorns and bay leaves.

SWEETCORN

Corn (maize) has been cultivated for 7–10,000 years, and adapted over many millennia to form the large cobs with its rows of tender grains (kernels) that we're familiar with today. It was a dietary staple of many early American cultures and, following its introduction to Europe in the sixteenth century, became an important crop that is now grown in almost every continent: along with soya, wheat and rice, it is one of the largest human food crops. Corn is processed to produce many products, and grown as a vegetable (though it is in fact a grass) and sold fresh, frozen or tinned. Sweetcorn cobs are succulent and sweet, but this sweetness fades quickly after harvesting, so eat them as soon as possible after purchase. If cobs are sold with husks intact, the husks should be clean and green, enclosing a cob with plump yellow kernels. Baby sweetcorn is picked when immature and has a milder flavour and a crunchy texture.

NUTRITIONAL BENEFITS
A good source of carotenes and vitamin A, B vitamins, vitamin C and iron.

SERVING SUGGESTIONS
Cook cobs in boiling water until tender (this can take anything from 5 to 15 minutes); add cooked or chargrilled kernels to a salsa, salad or tacos; add baby sweetcorn to stir-fries; add kernels to spiced vegetable fritter batters; stand fresh cobs upright on a chopping board, cut down to remove kernels, then add to a chowder; make a Mexican corn and black bean soup; peel the husks back from a cob (keeping them intact), then remove the silky threads, replace the husks, soak in cold water and cook slowly on the barbecue (wrap them in foil if they are husk-less); make a spiced corn relish with shallots and mustard seeds.

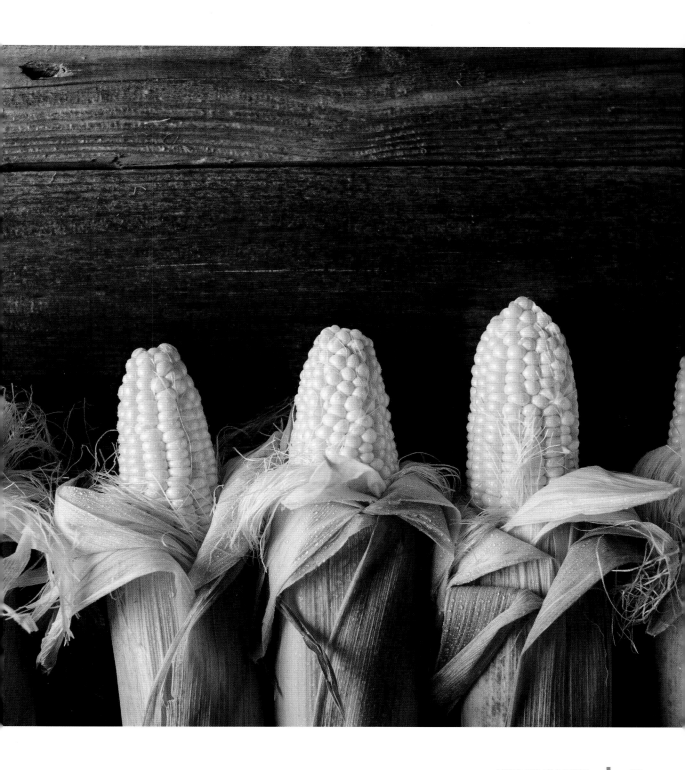

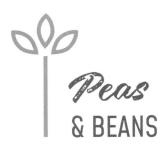

Peas
& BEANS

Peas and beans belong to the versatile and varied legume plant family and are among the oldest-known food crops. They have a high protein content – two or three times that of rice and wheat – and are very nutritious. The hundreds of varieties tend to fall into two groups: those with edible pods and those that need to be shelled. Most beans that require podding (such as flageolet and butter beans) are more commonly available in dried and tinned form. When buying fresh beans, firmness is a good indicator of freshness. Use well-salted water when cooking fresh beans and refresh them in cold water if you want to retain their vibrant colour.

PEAS

Native to west Asia, peas have been a staple food since ancient times. Dried peas were a key constituent of the European diet until, in the sixteenth century, a tender variety made for eating fresh was developed. Most modern-day pea production is still for dried peas, which are cooked whole, split or ground into flour. Peas cultivated for eating fresh are usually tinned or frozen within a few hours of picking. Frozen peas retain much of the sweetness that otherwise diminishes shortly after they are picked, and contain a higher nutritional content than fresh peas.

Petits pois are a dwarf variety of pea (not immature garden peas), and are particularly tender, with a sweet, delicate flavour.

NUTRITIONAL BENEFITS
Rich in calcium, magnesium, phosphorus, B vitamins, folic acid, potassium, zinc and iron.

SERVING SUGGESTIONS
Sauté an onion or spring onions in oil, add peas, shredded lettuce or cabbage and a little stock (or wine), cover and simmer until tender – serve as it is, or blitz to make a soup; make a pea risotto; add to an asparagus and broad bean salad; blitz to a purée with mint or coriander and serve as a dip; blanch and stir through bulgur wheat or other grain salad with fresh herbs.

MANGETOUT AND SUGAR SNAP PEAS

Fittingly, mangetout means 'eat everything' in French. These peas with edible pods are thought to have been first cultivated in the sixteenth century and there are two key types: flat-podded (mangetout or snow peas) and plump-podded (sugar snaps). The crunchy pods of both types contain rows of immature peas and are eaten whole. They have a delicate, sweet flavour and a crisp, tender texture (sugar snaps taste marginally sweeter than mangetout). Check for string on the edges of the pods before cooking, and remove if necessary. They should be small and crisp.

NUTRITIONAL BENEFITS
A good source of B vitamins, magnesium, phosphorus, potassium, vitamins A, C and K, folic acid and iron.

SERVING SUGGESTIONS
Steam or boil only briefly – for 1 or 2 minutes; add to a stir-fry; make a mangetout and mint soup; add whole mangetout or sugar snaps to a spring vegetable stew; blanch mangetout or sugar snaps and add to to a vibrant green bean, pea and herb salad; slice and stir into fried rice or noodles.

GREEN BEANS

Green edible-podded beans, now widely cultivated around the world, were first domesticated more than 5,000 years ago, and were introduced to Europe in the sixteenth century by explorers returning from the New World. Those grown for eating whole (as a vegetable), are known by many names, including common bean, French bean, haricot bean and string bean and are available fresh, tinned or frozen. The pods are mainly green, but can also be white, yellow, pink, violet or purple – the beans inside the pod can also vary in colour and shape. Early season beans can be eaten raw, though they are more commonly cooked. Round green beans are shorter and fatter than tender, slim French beans (*haricot verts*) which are harvested in the summer and are considered the cream of the crop in terms of taste and texture. All green beans should be firm and unblemished. For dried beans, see pages 92–7.

NUTRITIONAL BENEFITS
Fresh pods contain carotenes and vitamins B, C and E. The dried pulses contain 22 per cent protein and vitamins B and E.

SERVING SUGGESTIONS
Boil until just tender, then drain and serve warm or cold with a mustardy, garlicky vinaigrette; toss while warm with pesto or salsa verde; slowly stew French beans with softened onion and garlic, tomatoes and parsley until soft and tender and the tomato sauce is thick; chop green beans and stir-fry with oil, garlic and chilli; toss cooked beans into a vegan salad Niçoise.

RUNNER BEANS

The beans from this climbing plant are native to Central America and have been cultivated for more than 2,000 years. They were introduced to Britain in the fifteenth century, but initially found popularity as a decorative garden plant rather than a vegetable. They have a stronger flavour and more robust texture than French beans, and are larger, with long, flattened edible pods and rough-textured skin. They can be scarlet, green or white, and the beans in the pods can vary from pink to purple, to mottled dark. When they are very small, they can be eaten raw, but most require cooking to become tender. Runner beans should firm and bright green, and snap easily when you bend them. Avoid slicing them before cooking, as they will lose nutrients into the water. Top and tail before eating. Homegrown runner beans sometimes need stringing, though most cultivated varieties these days have stringless pods.

NUTRITIONAL BENEFITS

A good source of vitamins B, C and E and carotenes.

SERVING SUGGESTIONS

Boil or steam until tender; cook until tender, then toss in dressing while warm and serve with toasted nuts and croutons; shred and add to a tomato-based curry or Sri Lankan bean and coconut curry; braise with olive oil, onions, garlic and tomatoes until thickened and soft, then use to make filo pastry parcels, or serve on top of a bed of wild rice; make a runner bean chutney with onions, mustard, turmeric and vinegar.

BROAD BEANS

Before the discovery of the green beans of the New World, the only pulse available in Europe was the broad bean (also known as fava bean). It is native to Europe and was a vital source of protein in Europe, North Africa and the Middle East for millennia. It is now cultivated in temperate regions worldwide, and China produces much of the world's harvest. The largest of our commonly eaten legumes, broad beans vary in size and colour from white to green, to brown and have a meaty and mildly herbaceous flavour. When the beans in the pods are small and the pods are tender, the whole bean can be eaten whole (raw or cooked), but in most cases the beans are shelled from their tough pods, blanched then podded, or double-podded when large beans develop bitter skins. The older the bean, the stronger the flavour and the tougher their skins. Frozen broad beans retain much of their natural sweetness as they are frozen shortly after harvest.

NUTRITIONAL BENEFITS

A good source of vitamins A, B and C and contain carotenes.

SERVING SUGGESTIONS

Make the Egyptian stew, *ful medames* (the national dish of Egypt), with dried and soaked, tinned or fresh cooked broad beans, onion, herbs, spices and tomato passata; for a strong bean flavour, include broad bean pods in stocks for risottos and soups, removing them before serving; make broad bean, mint and courgette soup; add to fattoush (Middle Eastern toasted bread salad); blitz after shelling and boiling, with a little of the cooking water and some olive oil and herbs, to make a purée or dip; stir through cooked pasta; combine with baby artichokes and shallots in a risotto; add to a vegetable pilaf with other green beans; deep-fry young pods (after shelling) in batter and serve with dips.

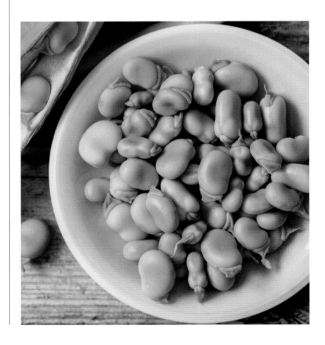

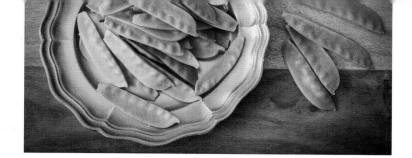

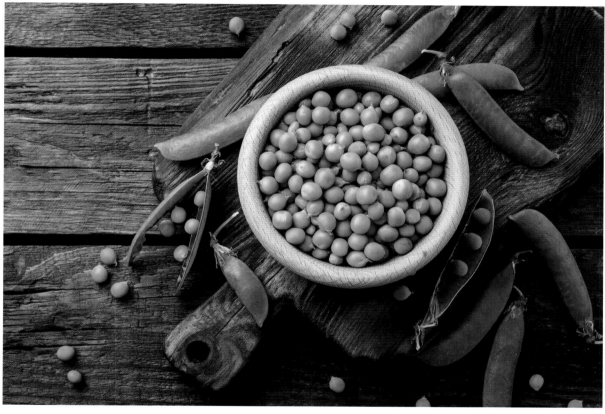

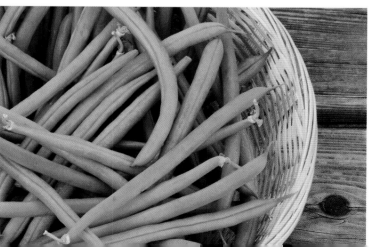

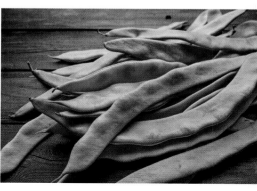

Sea vegetables

Sea vegetables have been harvested from our world's seashores and rocky coastlines for thousands of years. Rich in minerals and omega-3 fatty acids, edible ocean greens are cooked (fresh or rehydrated) and eaten as a succulent vegetable, or sold in dehydrated flakes, as powder or as compressed sheets, for use as a garnish or seasoning.

Carbohydrates extracted from seaweeds are used to thicken and stabilize ingredients instead of gelatine-based products, and algae-derived oils provide a vegan-friendly source of omega-3 fatty acids. Their iodine, umami flavour notes bring a taste of the sea to savoury dishes and are a key component of Japanese and Asian cuisines, where they are used in soups, stocks and as a component of sushi and onigiri.

SAMPHIRE:
There are two common types of samphire: marsh samphire and rock samphire. Marsh samphire grows in estuaries and salt marshes and is the most succulent of the two. Rock samphire grows on cliffs and rocks and is more resinous and stronger in taste.

KOMBU (ALSO KNOWN AS KONBU):
This variety of brown kelp grows off the coast of northern Japan. It is rich in MSG, and is a good source of iodine and selenium. It forms an essential element of the Japanese stock called dashi.

WAKAME:
Wakame looks similar to kombu and is popular in Japan and Korea. It has a mild, sweet flavour and can be toasted, crumbled and used as a condiment, or rehydrated and added to salads and soups.

NORI (LAVER):
Cultivated primarily in Japan, nori is the most widespread edible seaweed. A variety of red kelp, it is mostly widely available in dehydrated form, commonly in thin sheets. The sheets can be toasted to make them crisp and enable them to be easily crumbled into savoury dishes. Also known as laver, it has long been part of the Welsh and Irish diet. Welsh 'laverbread', boiled and puréed seaweed, is traditionally spread on bread and grilled, or rolled in oatmeal, then fried.

DULSE:
This succulent purple-red seaweed, dubbed the 'vegetarian oyster', is popular in Ireland, though it grows in both northern and southern hemispheres. It is typically soaked until soft, then added to soups, noodle dishes, salads and vegetable dishes.

CARRAGEEN (IRISH MOSS):
This reddish-purple seaweed with fan-shaped leaves is harvested primarily for the production of carrageenan, a stabilizing, gelling and emulsifying agent used in foods and cosmetic products.

AGAR-AGAR:
A gelling and thickening agent made from red marine algae, agar-agar is popular in Japan and tropical regions for making jellied confectionary and desserts, and adding to soups and sauces.

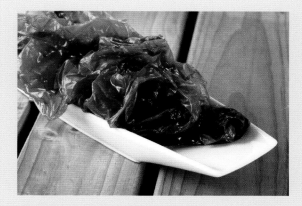

NUTRITIONAL BENEFITS
A rich source of iodine, protein, calcium, vitamins A, C, K, potassium and iron.

SERVING SUGGESTIONS
Scatter seaweed flakes over a noodle salad or stir-fry; add dried seaweed to stocks and broths; add crumbled, toasted nori to a tempura batter for vegetables or scatter over rice; make *norimaki* (seasoned rice wrapped in nori sheets); add fresh dulse or rehydrated wakame to a French onion soup or white bean purée; rehydrate wakame and use it as a base for a fried tofu salad; add seaweed flakes to crispbread or oatcake dough; use agar-agar as a setting agent in plant-based milk puddings such as panna cotta, trifle or blancmange; add rehydrated or fresh seaweed to potato rosti.

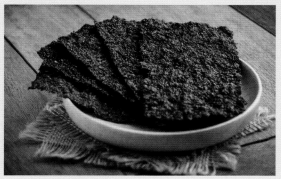

tip

Add a small strip of dried seaweed to the pan when cooking dried beans to help soften them and increase their digestibility.

Dried beans

Dried beans, an inexpensive and versatile staple in many cuisines, come in a vast range of sizes and colours and are a valuable source of protein, fibre and complex carbohydrates. Precooked beans are available tinned or frozen, and dried beans generally require rehydrating (by soaking then cooking) in order to become digestible – the soaking process reduces the cooking time. Dried beans are best cooked in just enough water to cover (which they will absorb during cooking), to avoid excessive loss of nutrients. Cook at a gentle simmer rather than a rolling boil (except dried kidney beans, which require initial hard boiling) for a more tender bean.

CHICKPEAS

Native to southwest Asia and Egypt and domesticated over 7,000 years ago, chickpeas are available in two types: smaller *desi* (common in Asia, Mexico and Ethiopia) and larger *kabuli* (common in the Middle East and Mediterranean). It is the most important legume in India, where it is known as *channa*. In India, chickpeas are often hulled and split to make channa dhal, or ground to a flour which is used to make savoury breads and pancakes. In the west, chickpeas are primarily used whole, either dried (and cooked) or tinned. They have a nutty flavour and smooth, buttery texture, and hold their shape well when cooked. Chickpeas contain less protein than most pulses, but more fat, and can be sprouted (see page 95).

NUTRITIONAL BENEFITS
A good source of iron, phosphorus and folic acid, calcium, magnesium, zinc, manganese and beta-carotene. High in fibre. Black chickpeas are more nutritious than white.

SERVING SUGGESTIONS
Blitz cooked chickpeas with cumin, lemon juice, olive oil and tahini to make a hummus; make falafel; stir cooked chickpeas through warm couscous or quinoa, with herbs and citrus, to make a salad; make a chickpea curry; roast until crispy, tossed with oil and a sprinkling of cayenne, paprika or cumin; simmer in a Moroccan vegetable stew or tagine.

KIDNEY BEANS

This variety of large-seeded common bean, native to the Andes, was the first to reach Europe (in the sixteenth century) and was given its name owing to its kidney shape. Kidney beans come in a range of colours, from white to red and black, though the most readily available in Europe are dark red. They are commonly associated with the Mexican dish, chilli con carne (Latin America is the largest consumer of the bean), and have a robust, full-bodied flavour and soft texture when cooked. The raw beans contain natural toxins called lectins, which are proteins that interfere with digestion and can prevent the intestine from absorbing nutrients. These are inactivated by high heat: after soaking dry beans, boil them vigorously for 20 minutes in fresh water, then cook slowly until tender (slow-cooking alone may mean they don't reach the required temperature to rid them of the toxins). Drain and rinse tinned beans before using.

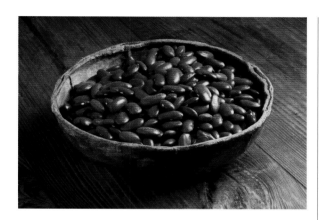

NUTRITIONAL BENEFITS
A good source of calcium, magnesium, phosphorus, potassium, folic acid and protein.

SERVING SUGGESTIONS
Add cooked beans to a bean casserole or salad; blitz cooked beans with grains, spices and herbs to make a bean burger; crush cooked beans, add spices to taste and serve with tacos, avocado and salsa; make Caribbean 'rice and peas', with onion, long-grain rice, coconut milk, tinned/cooked kidney beans and thyme.

CANNELLINI BEANS

This white bean, a member of the haricot bean family, is particularly popular in Italian cookery, where it appears in a multitude of rustic bean soups and stews, such as *pasta e fagioli*. The bean is larger and fatter than the haricot bean and has a mild, nutty flavour and smooth texture. When cooked, it takes on a pleasingly fluffy and soft texture. Cannellini beans are also known as Italian white

kidney beans or fasolia beans. The beans don't require soaking before cooking, but soaking will speed up the cooking process.

NUTRITIONAL BENEFITS
A good source of B vitamins, iron, potassium, calcium, zinc and other minerals.

SERVING SUGGESTIONS
Braise cooked beans in garlic and oil with stock or wine and herbs, then stir in wilted greens; cook and toss while still warm in a lemony dressing; make cannellini bean and leek soup; stew beans with sage and tomatoes; make an Iraqi-style stew (*fasoulia*) with cooked beans, tomatoes and baharat spice mix; blitz cooked beans with roasted garlic and oil to make a dip; pat dry tinned beans, then fry in oil until crispy.

FLAGEOLET BEANS

Another variety of haricot bean, these pale, green-white beans are available dried, semi-dried, fresh or tinned. Semi-dried (*demi-sec*) beans do not require soaking, just long cooking (45 minutes minimum). Flageolet beans are picked just before they are fully mature and are considered a particularly fine bean, with a tender, creamy texture and delicate, grassy flavour. They are used extensively in French cooking, particularly as fresh podded beans in casseroles, cassoulet and other slow-cooked dishes.

NUTRITIONAL BENEFITS
A good source of potassium, magnesium, iron, manganese, copper and vitamin B_9.

SERVING SUGGESTIONS
Slow-cook with tomatoes, garlic and oil; stir cooked beans through a vegetable or leaf salad; make a bean and pasta soup; toss cooked beans in a basil pesto.

BUTTER BEANS

These large, white beans (known as lima beans in the US – butter beans are the larger of two varieties of lima bean) originated in Peru and were transported to Europe and Africa in the sixteenth century, where they were adopted into western culinary culture, most notably in Spain and Greece. They have a rich, mellow flavour and soft, mealy texture and are flat and kidney-shaped. The large Judiones beans from northern Spain are particularly delicate and creamy. Baby butter beans are firmer and less buttery, and have a mild chestnut flavour.

NUTRITIONAL BENEFITS
Similar to the kidney bean. Rich in protein and a good source of potassium, calcium, phosphorus, magnesium, sodium, vitamin B_6 and iron.

SERVING SUGGESTIONS
Make a butter bean and tomato curry; blitz cooked beans with oil and herbs to make a smooth dip; stir through roasted root vegetables; blitz cooked beans with beetroot, bulghur wheat and onion to make falafel mixture, then fry in hot oil; add to a vegan gumbo; bake cooked beans with tomatoes, garlic and oil.

AZUKI BEANS

These small, russet-red beans, native to China, are the second most popular bean in Chinese, Korean and Japanese cookery (after soya beans). They have a mild, sweet, slightly nutty flavour and tender texture, and hold their shape well when cooked. In Japan, where they are prized as 'king of the beans', and in China, their natural sweetness is capitalized on and they are cooked and further sweetened to make a fresh bean paste used in confectionary. Azuki are small enough to cook without requiring soaking, and can be sprouted (see opposite).

NUTRITIONAL BENEFITS
A good source of protein, vitamin B_6, phosphorus, potassium, copper, magnesium, zinc and iron.

SERVING SUGGESTIONS
Make azuki bean burgers; 'pop' the beans, like corn kernels; make an azuki bean stew with onion, ginger, cinnamon and other warming spices and herbs; cook and stir through rice with sweet pickled cucumber; add to a vegan brownie mixture.

PINTO BEANS

This smaller, paler variety of the borlotti bean comes from the haricot bean family and has mottled red and white skin (pinto means 'speckled'). The beans have a mild, earthy flavour and creamy texture and can be cooked in a similar way to kidney or borlotti beans. They are a staple in North American, Brazilian and Mexican cooking and are the classic bean for Mexican refried beans, where the bean is cooked, then mashed and fried. In Northern Spain they are called *frijol pinto* ('speckled bean').

NUTRITIONAL BENEFITS
A good source of protein, phosphorus, folate, B vitamins and manganese.

SERVING SUGGESTIONS
Stew with peppers and tomatoes, with saffron, to make a Spanish-style bean stew, or stir them through a vegetable paella; stuff grilled peppers with cooked and mashed pinto beans mixed with grains and spices; add cooked beans to tacos and enchiladas.

BORLOTTI BEANS

This Italian variety of haricot bean, also called cranberry bean, is increasingly available in the west in its fresh form, as well as dried and tinned. The plump, oval beans grow in long pink-streaked pods and themselves have a mottled, pinkish skin (though they lose this attractive patterning when cooked and turn brown). Cooked borlotti beans have a sweet, nutty taste and creamy texture and, if simmered gently and slowly, hold their shape well. The beans don't require soaking before cooking, but soaking will speed up the cooking process.

NUTRITIONAL BENEFITS
A good source of protein, magnesium, phosphorus, potassium, copper, folate and manganese.

SERVING SUGGESTIONS
Add to a mixed bean salad; make Italian *pasta e fagioli*, a one-pot dish of fresh or dried and cooked borlotti, olive oil, garlic, rosemary, tomatoes and pasta; add tinned or cooked beans to minestrone soup; add to a vegetable stew or chilli; cook until tender, then roast with peppers and tomatoes; add to a beetroot soup or purin oile the beans and top with roasted beetroot.

HARICOT BEANS

Haricot is the generic name for fresh green beans in France, but in the UK and US it is the name for small ivory-white beans that are cultivated mainly to be sold dried or tinned. In the US they are called navy beans and they are the principle ingredient in the Boston baked beans dish, and they are the bean used for the ubiquitous tinned baked beans. The small, white plump beans retain their shape very well when they are cooked so are a perfect choice for slow-cooked recipes, and their mild flavour and buttery texture makes them particularly versatile.

NUTRITIONAL BENEFITS
A good source of B vitamins, folate, manganese, magnesium, iron and minerals.

Sprouting beans and lentils

Sprouting (germinating) beans and lentils is an ancient culinary tradition, particularly in Asia. Not only are sprouted beans and lentils highly nutritious, the process of activation also improves the bio-availability of the proteins and nutrients, and makes them more digestible. They are a rich source of vitamin C, and have a delicately nutty flavour and fresh, crunchy texture. Most whole beans and lentils, from tiny alfalfa seeds and azuki beans to chickpeas, soya beans and large broad beans, can be sprouted. Mung bean sprouts are the most well-known in the west, with soya bean sprouts coming a close second. Most can be eaten both raw and lightly cooked (soya bean and pinto bean sprouts should always be cooked). See page 116 for tips on activating nuts and seeds.

How to sprout beans or lentils at home:

1. Rinse and soak the beans or lentils in cold water for at least 12 hours until they swell. Rinse again.

2. Spread them out on a tray lined with clean muslin or thick kitchen paper. Store in a cool, dark place for 12 hours.

3. Rinse in a sieve under cold running water. Store in a cool, dark place on fresh clean muslin or paper for another 12 hours, or until the pale, green shoots are 1–2.5cm (½–1in) long. If shoots haven't yet appeared (chickpeas and black-eyed peas can take longer to germinate), repeat the rinsing and storing process at 12-hour intervals until they do.

4. Rinse again before eating, and keep in the fridge in a sealed container for up to 3–5 days.

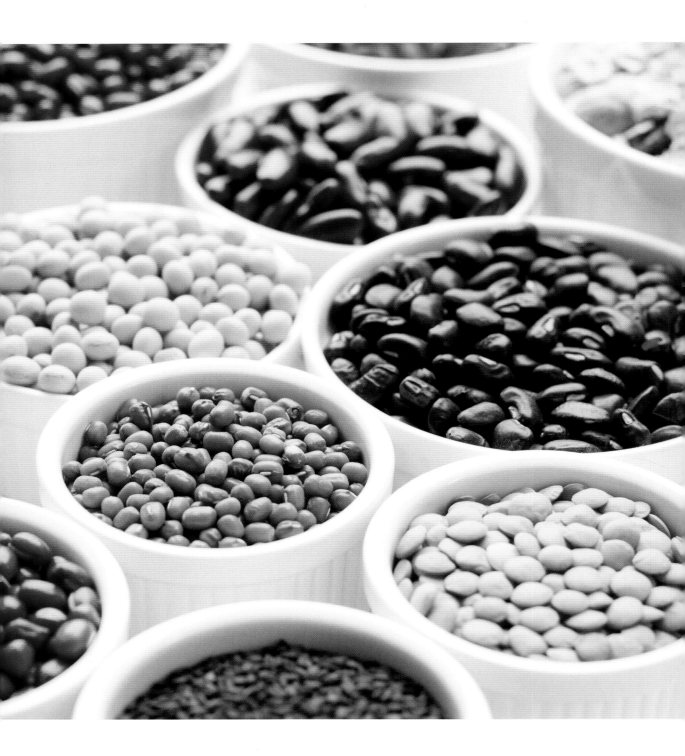

Stir cooked beans into a ratatouille; make home-made baked beans; use instead of chickpeas to make a hummus-style dip with tahini; add cooked beans to vegetable soups, stews or curries; mash cooked beans with oil; sauté spices in onion, garlic and oil, add rice and stock, cook until the rice is tender then, stir through cooked beans.

BLACK-EYED BEANS

This African relative of the mung bean is popular in South American Indian, Indonesian and African cuisines and is often served with rice. The small, ivory-coloured bean, also called cow pea and black-eyed pea, has a black mark where the bean was joined to the pod. They have a nutty, almost fruity taste, and a robust, chewy texture.

NUTRITIONAL BENEFITS
A rich source of calcium, folate and vitamin A.

SERVING SUGGESTIONS
Soak the beans, then cook with tomatoes, garlic and Moroccan spices to make a soup; cook, then blitz the beans with herbs, before frying to make Nigerian black bean fritters (*akara*); serve cooked beans with wilted spinach or chard; add cooked beans to a fresh tomato salsa; cook beans with spices, curry leaves, vegetable stock and coconut to make a curry; make a meat-free version of the Texan dish 'Hoppin' John', frying onion and celery, adding beans and rice, then stirring in herbs and cooking until tender.

BLACK BEANS

Native to Mexico, these black, shiny, oval-shaped beans are a staple food in Central and South America. Sometimes called turtle bean or *frijoles negros*, the beans are an essential ingredient in the national dish of Brazil, *feijoada*, and are a common side dish in Cuba. Their firm texture and earthy, rich flavour suits robust, strongly spiced dishes.

NUTRITIONAL BENEFITS
A rich source of iron, phosphorus, calcium, magnesium, manganese, folate, vitamin K, copper and zinc.

SERVING SUGGESTIONS
Add to a vegan moussaka or casserole; make black bean soup with cumin and coriander; fry in oil with garlic or onion, then stir through cooked rice or other grains and avocado, and serve as a salad or team with pickled onions and use to fill burritos; add to brownie batters.

MUNG BEANS

Mung beans are best known in their sprouted form (see page 95), but can also be bought whole, skinned or split. Originating in India (where they are sometimes known as green gram), mung have been widely used in Indian and Chinese cooking for thousands of years, and now grow throughout tropic and sub-tropic regions. One of the smallest dried beans, they are round, typically olive-green and have a slightly sweet, nutty flavour and creamy texture. Peeled and split mung beans are yellow.

NUTRITIONAL BENEFITS
A rich source of calcium, magnesium, iron, phosphorus, potassium, zinc, vitamins B_3 and B_5 and folic acid. Germination of the beans improved their nutritional qualities.

SERVING SUGGESTIONS
Add to a vegetarian chilli; cook moong dhal (split, skinned mung beans) with turmeric, cumin, garlic and chilli, and top with crispy fried shallots; cook soaked beans with onion, ginger, garlic, coconut milk and stock until the beans are cooked; toss cooked beans with roasted vegetables or fresh leaves and dress with a tahini and roasted lemon dressing.

Soya beans

Soya beans, domesticated in China since at least 3,000 BC and a staple food in China, Japan and Southeast Asia for millennia, were little known in the west until the nineteenth century. They are now the most widely consumed plant in the world. The fresh, immature beans have a very mild, fresh, pea-like flavour and crunchy texture when cooked, and are highly nutritious, containing all essential amino acids and double the protein content of many other legumes (about 35 per cent): this makes them particularly beneficial in regions where meat is rarely or never eaten.

The bean is also rich in oil (about 20 per cent in dried beans). Seed sizes vary, as do colours, which range from white to green, red, brown and black. The most common dried soya beans are small and pale brown.

A small proportion of the beans are grown as a fresh vegetable, picked when immature to be sold as edamame beans (popular in Japanese cuisine), but the majority of soya beans are harvested for the production of a wide range of foods and condiments, including tofu, fermented black beans, soy sauce, miso, tempeh and soy milk, made from the mature beans (green or black beans).

The process of transforming soya beans into these products 'unlocks' proteins and essential amino acids and increases their nutritional value. Mature soya beans are indigestible and bitter, so are not eaten in their natural state.

NUTRITIONAL BENEFITS

A rich source of calcium, iron, phosphorus, beta-carotene, amino acids, vitamin B_3, vitamins A, B and C, omega-3 essential fatty acids and protein. They supply almost as many essential amino acids as animal proteins and contain twice as much protein as other pulses.

SERVING SUGGESTIONS

Rub green soya bean pods with salt, then boil until tender before removing the beans from the pods (only the beans are edible); add cooked, podded beans to cooked brown or black rice with other vegetables and dress with soy sauce and sesame oil; crush cooked, podded beans and add to vegan burger mixtures; blend with a little miso to make a dip.

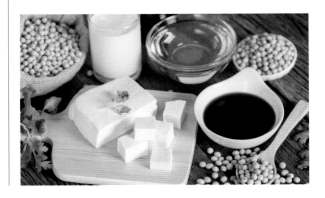

Soya bean products

MISO:

This salty fermented soya bean paste is integral to Japanese cuisine. Fermentation of the beans involves first growing a yeast mould (*koji*) on steamed grains (usually rice, though barley or rye are also sometimes used), then soaking, steaming and chopping the beans before combining them with the mould, grains, salt and water that has had yeast and bacteria cultures added to it. The mixture is then left to ripen. The range of colours in miso products is due to the varied ingredients and methods of fermentation: typically, the greater the amount of rice used, and the shorter the fermentation time, the lighter (and sweeter) the miso.

White miso is pale-yellow, milder, and less salty than red or brown misos. Good-quality, traditionally-made miso has a strong, complex and distinctive savoury (umami) taste. *Doenhang* soya bean paste is a Korean style of miso that has a coarser consistency and stronger flavour. Miso is rich in minerals and vitamin B_{12}. Add it to stock, make a miso marinade for tofu or vegetables destined for the oven or grill, or add to salad dressings and noodle dishes.

SOY SAUCE :

This salty condiment is made of fermented soya beans. Originally it was a paste rather than a sauce, until the excess liquid from the paste became more popular than the paste itself. According to traditional production methods, soy sauce is made by steaming soya beans, then mashing them with roasted, crushed wheat (the proportion of wheat and soya beans varies according to the style being made). A starter culture is added, the mixture starts fermenting, then salt is added, along with another starter culture, with fermentation and maturation continuing for 8–12 months. The mixture is filtered to extract the sauce, which is then pasteurized and bottled before being used as a condiment and flavour enhancer, and in cooking. The darker the sauce, the longer it has been aged. Use soy sauce as a dipping sauce for spring rolls, wontons and vegan sushi, or add to stir-fries, sauces and marinades.

Japanese white soy sauce: made with a higher percentage of wheat than traditional soy sauce, white soy sauce is prized in Japan for its pale colour and delicate flavour. In Japan, light soy sauces are preferred to dark.

Light soy sauce: this Chinese soy sauce has a thinner texture than dark soy sauce. It is made from the first pressing of the fermented soya beans and is saltier than dark.

Dark soy sauce: another Chinese soy sauce, this is aged longer than light soy sauce, and has a thicker texture and richer, sweeter taste.

NATTO:

A quick-fermented Japanese product made of cooked soya beans that are fermented for about 20 hours. It has a strong, musty flavour and sticky and slimy, stringy texture. It is served with rice and noodles, in salads and soups, or cooked with vegetables.

TEMPEH:

An Indonesian speciality, tempeh is a thin cake made with quick-fermented, unsalted soya bean curds. It is similar to tofu but has a more savoury and mushroomy flavour that becomes nutty when it's cooked. Whole, dry soya beans are soaked until soft, partially de-hulled, then boiled and drained before a starter culture is added and the beans are left to ferment for about 24 hours (the longer they are left to ferment (ripen), the stronger the flavour). Tempeh can also be made with other beans, grains and seeds. It plays a crucial nutritional role in the rice-based diet of the Javanese. Use it in the same way as tofu.

TOFU:

Tofu is made by soaking dried yellow soya beans in water, grinding and boiling them, then filtering them to produce soya milk. A coagulating agent (called *nigari* in Japan) is then added, to make it curdle. The warm curds are pressed to squeeze out the 'whey', a process similar to that used in cheese-making.

The various consistencies of tofu can be considered as alternatives to their dairy counterparts in all manner of dishes. Relatively tasteless, its merits lie in its rich nutritional properties and its versatility in the kitchen. It is an excellent source of protein, and is rich in iron, amino acids, potassium, calcium, magnesium and vitamins A and K.

Soft/silken tofu: silken tofu consists of unpressed, uncurdled milk and has a delicate, custard-like texture. Chinese silken tofu is softer and eaten hot or cold, with a spoon rather than sliced. It is well suited to both sweet and savoury dishes. Use as a soft cheese/dairy replacement in baked savoury dishes such as a vegan lasagne, to make dips, or in puddings, ice creams and smoothies.

Plain/semi-pressed white tofu: the curds are pressed so the tofu holds its shape and can be sliced or diced, and packaged in water.

This is most widely available type of tofu. Commonly used in soups and braised dishes, or fried until it puffs up.

Firm tofu: firm tofu has more water pressed from it, and is firmer than plain tofu, with a creamy, smooth texture. It is sold in blocks, packaged in water. Drain and pat dry before using. Cube or slice and deep-fry, marinate cubed tofu and add to soups and stir-fries, or serve cold in salads.

Smoked tofu: firm tofu that has been smoked. The smoking process browns the surface, but the tofu remains white inside. Slice or dice and add to stir-fried greens, serve with noodles or cold dishes.

Freeze-dried tofu: freeze-dried tofu has a spongy, chewy texture and doesn't fall apart when cooked. It needs to be reconstituted with water before using.

Fermented tofu: Also called fermented bean curd, the two most widely available forms are red or white (the red style is often made with chillies). It is made with dried, fermented tofu that is then soaked in brine or rice wine. It is smooth, soft and spreadable, and is typically added to braised dishes, rice porridge and stir-fries. Use sparingly.

For soy milk see page 103.

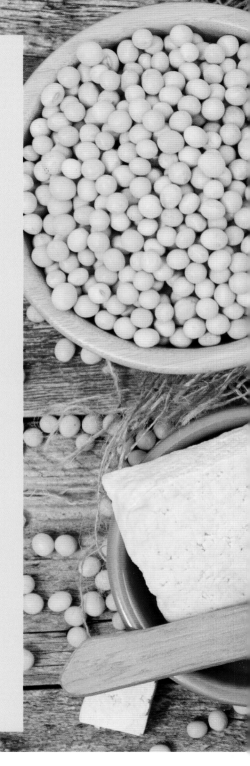

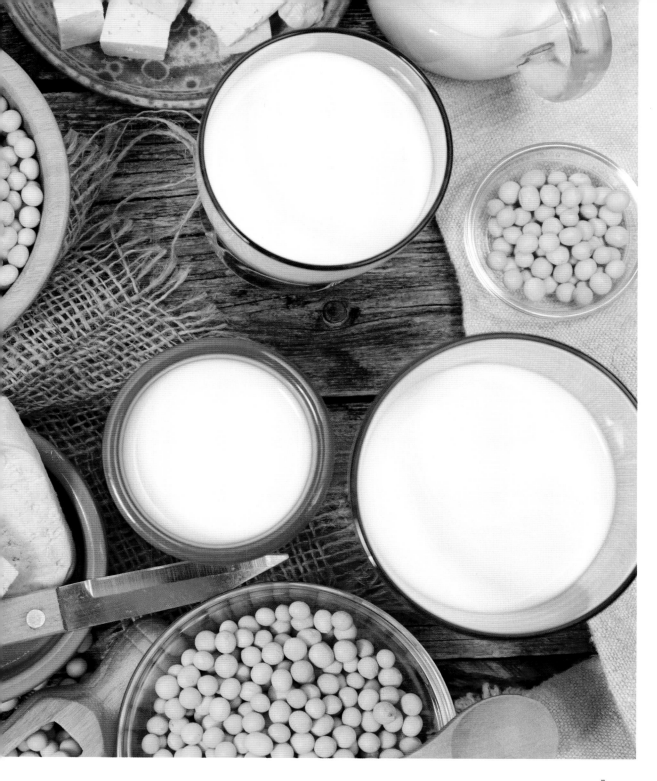

Vegan milks

Plant-based milks are made by soaking and grinding cooked or heat-treated nuts, seeds, beans or grains, then blending them with water. They contain less calcium and protein than diary milk, so ensure you're eating foods rich in calcium, iodine and protein to avoid a deficiency. Most plant-based milks are available sweetened or unsweetened and many are fortified with minerals and vitamins such as B, D and calcium.

OAT MILK

Made from oat groats (cleaned, hulled and toasted oats) and water. Oat milk contains more B vitamins than soy and coconut milk and more protein than almond milk, and is often fortified with added calcium. It is an ideal non-dairy milk option for anyone with a nut allergy. Oat milk has a higher fibre content than other non-dairy milks, in the form of soluble beta-glucan.

PEA MILK

An increasingly popular non-diary drink made from milled yellow field peas. Pea milk is naturally high in protein, and has a flavour and consistency not unlike cow's milk.

ALMOND MILK

One of the most popular non-dairy milks, almond milk has a mild, nutty flavour, though technically it is a seed, not a nut. It typically consists of 2–6 per cent almonds, water, salt (and sometimes sweetener), thickeners and added vitamins D and E. It contains phytic acid (as does soy milk), which can inhibit the body's absorption of iron and other minerals, so consume it at least 30 minutes before or after consuming iron-rich foods. It is low in fat and protein, but many manufacturers fortify their products with extra protein. Other nut milks include cashew (creamier than almond milk), hazelnut and peanut milks.

COCONUT MILK DRINK

Made from the white flesh of the coconut, which is pulverized, filtered and blended with water. Coconut milk has higher saturated fat (and higher calorie) content than most plant-based milks and a sweet taste. It contains fibre, potassium and iron, but almost no protein. Don't confuse coconut milk drinks with 'coconut milk', which is thicker and sold in tins for cooking and desserts.

HEMP MILK

Made from the hulled seeds of the hemp plant, hemp milk has an earthier flavour and contains more plant-based fatty acids than most non-dairy milks and is often enriched with calcium and vitamin D. It is a good dairy alternative for anyone with a nut or soya allergy, though it's lower in protein than soy milk.

SOY MILK

Prepared from steamed, pressed soya beans, soy milk is rich in protein and iron but low in fat and carbohydrates. Nutritionally, of all the non-dairy milks it's the closest equivalent to cow's milk, though it contains less calcium, iodine and B vitamins so these are often added in the production process. It can be bought in powdered form to add to smoothies and other beverages to boost protein intake. Probiotic and fermented soy milks are also available. Look for products that list whole soya beans in their ingredients lists rather than 'soy protein isolate' or 'isolated soy protein'.

RICE MILK

Made from ground rice and water, most rice milks are fortified with calcium and vitamin D. Grain milks are slightly higher in natural sugars, due to the grain's carbohydrates, so are naturally sweeter than most non-dairy milks (and not recommended for diabetics). Rice milk is a good beverage for anyone with a nut or soya allergy. Look for brands made with whole brown rice rather than rice protein. Less widely available grain milks include quinoa milk and spelt milk. For a rice milk recipe, see page 161.

Understanding additives on a nut or grain milk label

GUAR GUM
Derived from the seed of the guar plant, used a thickener and binding agent.

GELLAN GUM
An artificially produced soluble fibre, used as a thickener and stabilizer.

LOCUST BEAN/CAROB BEAN GUM
Derived from the seed of the carob tree, and used as a thickener.

TAPIOCA STARCH
Powdered cassava plant used as a thickener.

CARRAGEENAN
An additive derived from red seaweed, used as a thickening and emulsifying agent.

PEA PROTEIN
Dried extract of yellow or green peas, used to boost protein content of non-diary milks.

D-ALPHA-TOCOPHEROL
Vitamin E.

CALCIUM PHOSPHATES / CALCIUM CARBONATE
Mineral derived from chalk, plants or/and ammonia, used to boost calcium content in non-dairy milks.

NUTRITIONAL YEAST
See box on page 155.

MALTODEXTRIN
A sweetener derived from potato or corn.

DI-POTASSIUM PHOSPHATE / ACIDITY REGULATOR
Salt derived from phosphate rock.

CHICORY ROOT FIBRE (SOMETIMES CALLED INULIN)
A carbohydrate fibre that mimics the creaminess of animal fat.

SUNFLOWER LECITHIN
A gum substance derived from dehydrated sunflower, used as a stabilizer and source of fatty acids.

POTASSIUM CITRATE
A mixture of potassium salt and citric acid, used to regulate acidity.

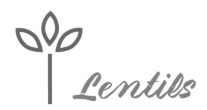

Lentils

This nourishing, economical ingredient is thought to be the oldest of the cultivated legumes. Domesticated over 8,000 years ago in southwest Asia, these dried seeds of pod-bearing plants come in a full spectrum of colours and have long been a staple food, particularly in India, the Mediterranean and the Middle East. They are a key source of protein in the vegetarian diets of the Indian subcontinent, and are rich in fibre, vitamin B_g, iron and phosphorus. Whole lentils can be bought pre-cooked (tinned or in pouches) and dried, and split lentils (husked or unhusked) are sold dried. Whole lentils take longer to cook than split lentils. Lentils can also be sprouted (see page 95).

GREEN AND BROWN LENTILS

Larger than split lentils, disc-shaped green and brown lentils feature in a number of European cuisines, particularly in hearty savoury dishes and soups. They both have a mildly nutty, earthy flavour and can be used interchangeably, but should be cooked gently in order to retain their shape and firm texture: these lentils have a tendency to disintegrate more easily than Puy lentils. Cook them for about 20 minutes (older lentils might take longer). Although whole lentils don't need to be soaked, soaking does help make the nutrients in the lentils more accessible, and enables them to be more easily digested (soak green and brown lentils for 8–10 hours, or overnight).

NUTRITIONAL BENEFITS
A good source of calcium, magnesium, phosphorus, potassium, zinc and folic acid, and vitamins A and B.

SERVING SUGGESTIONS
Make a squash and lentil soup; add cooked lentils to a vegan burger mixture; cook, then mash roughly to make a dip and scatter with Egyptian dukkah; make Middle Eastern koshari, a dish of rice cooked with lentils, garlic and onions, served with a spiced tomato sauce; add to a vegan shepherd's pie; make a lentil, coconut and tomato soup; add cooked lentils to a lemony potato and spinach or chard soup.

PUY LENTILS

These slate-green speckled lentils are grown in the fertile, volcanic soil of the Auvergne region of France. They are smaller than green or brown lentils, hold their shape better when cooked, and are renowned for their delicate, rich earthy flavour, which has a mildly peppery bite (they are known locally as the 'caviar of the poor'). Their desirability is reflected in their price. Puy lentils cook in 25–40 minutes and are typically served alone, dressed in vinaigrette, and in salads.

NUTRITIONAL BENEFITS
A good source of calcium, magnesium, phosphorus, potassium, zinc and folic acid, and vitamins A and B.

SERVING SUGGESTIONS
Braise with onion, wine and herbs; add cooked lentils to a vegetable lasagne or gratin; combine cooked lentils with roasted vegetables – such as beetroot, onion aubergine or red pepper – and smoked or marinated, fried tofu cubes; combine with pea shoots, watercress or charred broccoli

in a green salad; toss warm cooked lentils in a mustardy vinaigrette; add to a warm bean or roasted carrot salad; use to make a lentil ragu or combine with beans and smoked paprika in a hearty chilli.

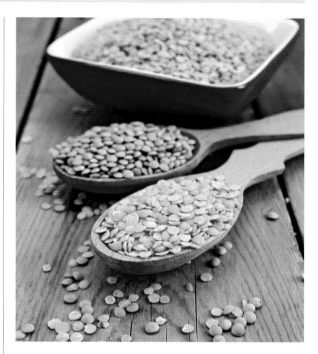

RED SPLIT LENTILS

Also known as the Egyptian split lentil or masoor dhal, this husked split pulse is key to one of the Indian subcontinent's principle dishes – dhal ('dhal' is the Hindi term for split lentils, peas and other dried pulses, and the name for the cooked dish). The small lentils can be pale orange, deep orange or red (this colour fades during cooking) and have a mild flavour that works well with strong spices. When cooked, the lentils quickly disintegrate so are best suited to soups, curries and used as a thickener. They don't require soaking and cook in 15–20 minutes. Rinse before cooking.

Yellow split lentils taste similar to red split lentils and can be cooked in the same way, and they have a unique, subtle sweetness and nuttiness.

NUTRITIONAL BENEFITS
A good source of calcium, magnesium, phosphorus, potassium, zinc and folic acid, and vitamins A and B.

SERVING SUGGESTIONS
Simmer in water or stock; make curried lentil soup; cook with spices to make a dhal and top with crispy fried onions or tarka (spices fried in oil); combine with spices and vegetables (roast squash works well) to make kofte or shami kebabs, then fry; use to thicken soups and stews; make a spiced red lentil and cumin dip.

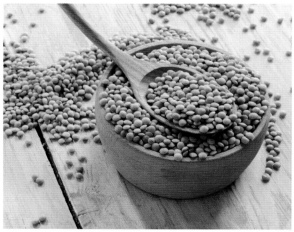

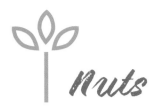

Nuts

Nut-bearing trees are one of the world's oldest food plants. Nuts (the dried tree fruits) are highly nutritious and rich in fat, B vitamins, vitamin E and minerals. Some nuts are available fresh ('green'), but most are dried, and they are all versatile ingredients, suiting both sweet and savoury uses. Ground and chopped nuts are often added to savoury dishes and cakes, and whole nuts are eaten as snacks, and used for decorating and flavouring bakes and confectionary. Nuts are also made into flour, oil, butter and milk products (see page 102). Buy nuts in small quantities and store in an airtight container in a cool place. Toasting nuts emphasizes their nuttiness.

PEANUTS

Peanuts, technically a legume, originated in South America, coming to Europe with the return of the explorers of the New World and quickly finding popularity in tropical and sub-tropical regions the world over. The bushy plant pushes its nut-bearing pods into the ground to mature, after it has flowered. Peanuts are a staple protein-rich food in Southeast Asia and west Africa, used largely in savoury dishes such as soups, stews and sauces, and in the west are more commonly eaten as a snack food or as peanut butter. They are also known as groundnuts. India and China are the main producers of peanuts (primarily for the nut oil), followed by the USA (for the whole nut).

Peanuts can be bought in the shell, shelled but raw, roasted skinned and roasted unskinned.

NUTRITIONAL BENEFITS
Contain more protein than most nuts (20–30 per cent), are high in fat and rich in fibre, iron, folate and niacin, and vitamin A.

SERVING SUGGESTIONS
Make nut butter (see page 162); make satay sauce by blitzing unsalted peanut butter (or roasted unsalted peanuts ground to a crumb) with water or coconut milk, soy sauce, lime juice, garlic and rice vinegar and sugar to taste; use peanut butter in vegan cookies; add roasted peanuts to a tofu and broccoli pad thai; combine peanut butter and fruit jelly in vegan brownies; use peanut butter instead of tahini in baba ganoush (aubergine dip) or hummus; toss roasted, unsalted peanuts through a cold Chinese noodle salad.

CASHEW NUTS

These seeds come from the fruit of the Brazilian tropical 'cashew apple' tree. When the nut (fruit) reaches maturity on the tree, a large pear-like 'fruit' expands between the nut and the branch and when the fruit is ripe, the kidney-shaped nut falls to the ground. The fruit is eaten raw, cooked, or made into jam, juice or wine in countries where cashews are grown. It is difficult to extract the nuts from their shells, and the shells contain irritants, so nuts are sold shelled (raw or roasted). The tree is native to South America though cashews are now widely grown throughout tropical regions. They have a buttery texture and a mild flavour that's sweeter than most nuts. In South India and China they are used whole or ground in savoury dishes. Elsewhere, they tend to feature more frequently in sweet dishes. They are sold whole, halved or chopped.

NUTRITIONAL BENEFITS
High in fat (but lower than almonds, peanuts, pecans and walnuts) and a good source of essential fatty acids, carbohydrate, B vitamins, calcium, copper, magnesium, iron, zinc and folic acid.

SERVING SUGGESTIONS
Make nut butter (see page 162); toss with spices and oil and roast in the oven; toss toasted cashews through fried rice or stir-fried vegetables; add chopped, toasted cashews to the base of a sweet no-bake vegan cheesecake; add to a Sri Lankan butternut squash and coconut-milk curry or Indian korma; stir toasted nuts through a brown rice pilaf; soak raw nuts in water overnight, then use as a vegetable in a coconut-based Goan-style curry.

PISTACHIO NUTS

These striking pale- or bright-green nuts with a thin, reddish-purple skin come from a small tree native to Central Asia. The nut is the kernel of the stone of a small fruit which resembles an olive and grows in clusters. Pistachios have long been a familiar and prized feature of Middle Eastern Mediterranean and Turkish cuisines. They have a mild but distinctive flavour and creamy texture and are sold shelled or in a split shell (the shells are easy to open) – the darker green the nut, the more highly prized it is. Pistachios are eaten as a snack and used in myriad sweet and savoury dishes, from ice creams, nougat and halva to savoury terrines and rice dishes, and as a garnish for confectionary.

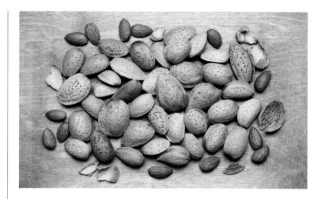

NUTRITIONAL BENEFITS
A very rich source of potassium and iron, they also contain calcium, magnesium, vitamin A and folate.

SERVING SUGGESTIONS
Make a vivid green, coarse pistachio nut butter (see page 162) then combine it with syrup, rose water or orange water and use it to make crisp filo-pastry parcels; make halva with maple syrup, pistachios and tahini; scatter over, or stir through, a butternut squash and saffron pilaf; combine chopped unsalted pistachios with spices to make Egyptian dukkah to use for dipping or scattering over vegetables or salads; make a pistachio pesto; make pistachio and dark chocolate florentines.

ALMONDS

Almonds are the most popular nut in the world. One of the earliest domesticated nut trees, they have been cultivated since classical times in warm, temperate regions, and were much loved by the ancient Romans and Greeks. They belong to the same family of trees as the plum, cherry, apricot and peach, but the leathery fruit that contains the nut (seed) can only be eaten when immature. Two varieties are cultivated: sweet and bitter. Bitter almonds are grown for almond oil, extract and liqueurs, and sweet almonds for eating. The kernel within the narrow, oval shell has a mild, milky and delicate taste and is covered by brown skin, which is sometimes intact, sometimes removed by blanching. Almonds are available whole, split, flaked, chopped or ground. They are widely used in Middle Eastern cuisines and in the making of southern European pastries and Spanish confectionary, and are the main ingredient in marzipan, a paste of sugar and finely ground almonds. They can be eaten raw or cooked – roasting them gives them a richer taste.

NUTRITIONAL BENEFITS
High in monounsaturated fats, a good source of protein, vitamins B_2 and E, iron and zinc. The second highest source of vitamin E after hazelnuts, and the richest nut source of calcium.

SERVING SUGGESTIONS
Add ground almonds to cake batters and pastry doughs; scatter vegetable and couscous salad or a spiced tagine with toasted flaked almonds; make almond and hazelnut butter (see page 162); toast flaked almonds and sprinkle over French beans or asparagus in vinaigrette; use blanched almonds in the Spanish cold soup *ajo blanco*; add almond butter to a cherry smoothie; add toasted almonds to Italian panforte, the rich Tuscan fruit and nut cake; use almond butter in a sweet and spicy miso-based sauce for noodles, salad or roasted vegetables; toast with rosemary to serve as a snack.

HAZELNUTS

These small nuts with hard brown shells come from the fruit of bushy hazel trees and have been cultivated in Europe and other temperate regions for many thousands of years – evidence suggests they were being eaten during the Bronze Age. They have a rich and buttery flavour and a lower oil content than most nuts. In Britain, sweet, fresh hazelnuts (known as cobnuts) are an autumn speciality: they have a pale, green-brown shell and crunchy, milky flesh. Most hazelnuts, however, are mature nuts that are sold raw or roasted, shelled, unshelled or ground. Those grown in the Piedmont region of Italy are considered particularly fine. Hazelnuts of a slightly different variety are known in the US as filberts. If you prefer to remove their thin, papery skin, roast them for a few minutes in the oven until light brown, then rub the skins off with a tea towel. The producers of a certain chocolate-nut spread use 25 per cent of the world's hazelnut supply.

NUTRITIONAL BENEFITS
A rich source of magnesium, B vitamins and copper and particularly rich in vitamin E.

SERVING SUGGESTIONS
Add ground, toasted hazelnuts to a carrot cake mixture; fold roasted, chopped hazelnuts into aquafaba meringue mixture before baking; make hazelnut butter with roasted hazelnuts and cocoa (see page 162); make the Catalonian paste *picada* with pounded hazelnuts, garlic, toasted bread and oil, and use to pep up vegetable stews, braises or serve as a dip; make a hazelnut romesco sauce with red peppers; toast and chop, then sprinkle over pasta dishes or green beans; add to granola.

WALNUTS

Large walnut trees grow wild in temperate regions and have been cultivated widely for their oil-rich nuts for thousands of years. Green tree-fruit surround the stone, which contains half-kernels separated by a bitter, papery membrane. The English walnut, also known as the Persian walnut, is the most widely available variety. The mature nuts have a mild, sweet flavour with a pleasantly astringent tang and are sold in the shell, shelled, chopped or ground. Young, fresh walnuts are called 'wet' walnuts, and their pale, sweet creamy flesh can be eaten raw in the late autumn-winter (though they are more often salted or pickled in spiced vinegar). Black walnuts, cultivated in North America, have a very dark brown shell and a more assertive, fruitier taste. Walnuts suit both sweet and savoury cooking, from cakes and biscuits to soups, dressings and stews.

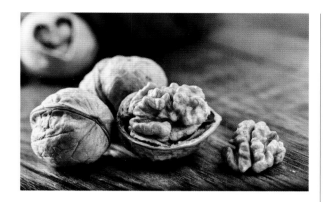

NUTRITIONAL BENEFITS

Rich in vitamins, especially folate, plus magnesium, potassium, iron and zinc. Also high in omega-3 fatty acids.

SERVING SUGGESTIONS

Use instead of pine nuts in pesto; toast and blitz with vegan milk/water-soaked bread, garlic, olive oil and lemon juice to make a dip; scatter roasted walnuts over a couscous and roasted beetroot salad; fold roasted walnuts into bread dough; stir roasted, chopped nuts into caramel, sprinkle with black pepper and leave to set to make a sweet brittle; make Persian aubergine *fesenjan*, with aubergine, walnuts and pomegranate molasses.

PECAN NUTS

This oil-rich nut is native to America and was a staple food for North American Indians before the arrival of Europeans. The large tree on which it grows comes from the same plant family as the walnut. Pecan nuts resemble walnuts – both nuts come in two halves – but are sweeter and oilier than walnuts and do not share their astringency. The tender nut is formed inside a smooth, thin yet brittle shell with a pointed tip and can be bought unshelled and raw, shelled and raw, or roasted and salted. They are primarily used in sweet dishes such as cookies and cakes, particularly in America (its most well-known use is the southern American Thanksgiving speciality, pecan pie), but their buttery, mild sweetness works well in savoury dishes too.

NUTRITIONAL BENEFITS

Rich in vitamins A and B$_1$, fibre, iron, calcium, copper, magnesium, potassium and phosphorus. High in fats (they contain more fat than any other nut).

SERVING SUGGESTIONS

Toast and scatter over salads; to candy the nuts, pan-fry with equal quantities of water and sugar, and the zest of an orange, until the water has evaporated and the nuts are caramelized; add chopped pecans to sweet or savoury bread dough or to date energy balls; scatter over vegan blueberry or blackberry pancakes; toss roasted diced sweet potato with pecans and maple syrup; combine with vegan butter, sugar and oats, then use as a crumble topping for grilled nectarines or peaches.

MACADAMIA NUTS

Macadamia nuts come from a subtropical evergreen tree native to the woodlands of Australia. They were eaten by indigenous Australians for thousands of years before being introduced to the Americas in the late 1800s. They flourished in Hawaii, which – with Australian and South Africa – now produces much of the world's supply of macadamias. The nuts grow in clusters, in thick and fleshy green husks. When fully mature, they fall to the ground and the husks split open to expose the nuts in their shells, which are then harvested and shelled. These shells are extremely hard and the trees take many years to bear fruit, which makes macadamias a pricey nut. They are pale gold and have a sweet, delicate flavour and rich, buttery texture and are more popular for snacking than as a cooking ingredient.

NUTRITIONAL BENEFITS

A good source of B vitamins and minerals including thiamine and magnesium. They contain 66 per cent oil and are the fattiest nut after pecans.

SERVING SUGGESTIONS

Add unsalted macadamias to granola before baking; chop unsalted macadamias finely and add to vegan burger or nut roast mixtures along with mushrooms; add unsalted macadamias to biscotti dough; toss unsalted nuts in maple syrup, oil and spices and bake until sticky and caramelized; make macadamia brittle, to serve with desserts; purée with water and strain to make nut milk (see page 161).

BRAZIL NUTS

These large nuts come from the fruit of a giant tree that grows wild in the rainforests of Brazil and surrounding Amazon regions. The nuts grow in groups of eight to twenty-four, tightly packed together in their own woody casings within a large brown coconut-sized fruit, which falls to the ground from high up in the canopy when ripe (harvesting them is a dangerous business). They are sold shelled and unshelled, raw or roasted and salted, and have a sweet, milky taste and creamy, waxy texture.

Their high oil content (up to 65 per cent) means they go rancid more rapidly than other nuts, so buy them in small quantities and use quickly once opened.

NUTRITIONAL BENEFITS
Rich in protein, iron, calcium, B vitamins, vitamin A and zinc. Brazil nuts contain the highest natural source of selenium – one nut exceeds the recommended RDA.

SERVING SUGGESTIONS
Chop and fry with Brussels sprouts; scatter cakes and biscuits with chopped brazil nuts before baking; add to a savoury nut crumble for roasted vegetables or sweet crumble for desserts; make a brazil nut pesto and serve with roasted vegetables or pasta; add toasted nuts to a pilaf or black bean burger mixture.

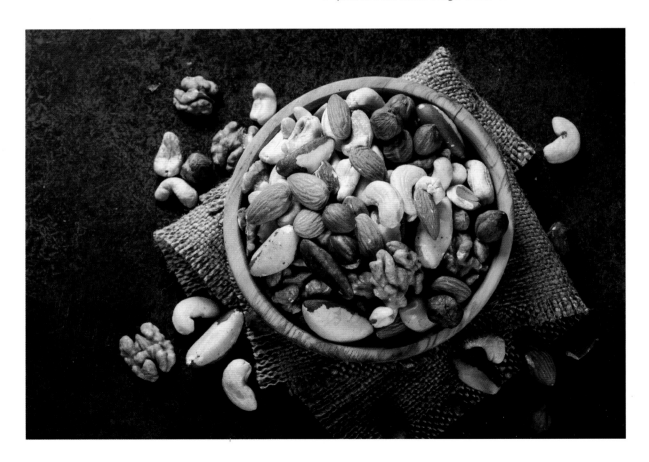

CHESTNUTS

Native to temperate West Asia, the large sweet chestnut tree was brought to southern Europe by the Greeks, where it thrived and was used in cooking as a flour and a nut. Cultivated chestnuts produce a single nut in each prickly bur (nut-case) that looks similar to the horse chestnut (an important difference: the horse chestnut's fruit and seeds are inedible). They have a soft, floury texture and sweet, nutty flavour and should not be eaten raw. Fresh chestnuts are sometimes sold in late autumn and winter with glossy brown skins intact, for the purpose of roasting, which emphasizes their earthy sweetness. Before roasting, a small cross or hole should be cut in the shell to prevent them exploding. Peel away the tough skin and papery inner skin while still warm. Cooked and ready-peeled chestnuts in vacuum-packed pouches make a convenient alternative to fresh chestnuts. They are also sold as a sweetened purée for using in desserts, and as marrons glacés (chestnuts soaked in syrup). Chestnut flour is used in Italy to thicken savoury dishes and in baking.

NUTRITIONAL BENEFITS
A good source of minerals and potassium. Contain less oil and protein than most other nuts, and more starch.

SERVING SUGGESTIONS
Scatter fresh roasted chestnuts over a risotto; make chestnut and butternut squash or parsnip soup; use freshly ground, roasted chestnuts in cake mixtures; make a savoury, herby crumble with chestnuts and rosemary for sprinkling over soups and salads; blitz cooked chestnuts with a little water to make a purée and add to salad dressings; fry cooked chestnuts with mushrooms; mix chopped cooked chestnuts with dried fruit, cocoa and spices and use as a sweet pastry filling.

PINE NUTS

These small cream-coloured seeds come from the cones of about twelve species of the evergreen pine tree: the seeds form at the base of the scales which form the pine cones. The slender, elongated seeds of the European Stone Pine are the most highly prized and are richer in oil than the more common pine nuts from northern Asia. Pine nuts, also called pine kernels, feature frequently in the cuisines of the Middle East – where they have been used for millennia – and the Mediterranean. They are key ingredient in Italian Genoese basil pesto and the Middle Eastern sauce, *tarator* (this also works well with walnuts), and appear frequently in the cakes and bakes of Sicily and Malta. Their soft texture and subtle, slightly resinous flavour becomes rich, sweet and aromatic when the nuts are gently toasted. Toast carefully, as their high oil content means they easily burn.

NUTRITIONAL BENEFITS
A good source of protein, calcium, magnesium, potassium, zinc and B vitamins.

SERVING SUGGESTIONS
Combine with spinach for a ravioli filling or pasta sauce with griddled courgettes; combine with basil or other soft green herbs to make pesto; scatter toasted pine nuts over a pilaf before serving; scatter over the Turkish dish of aubergine baked with onions and tomatoes (*imam bayildi*); sprinkle toasted pine nuts over a roasted tomato tart; roll chocolate truffles in roughly chopped or whole toasted pine nuts.

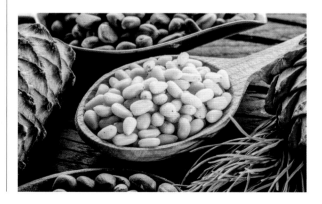

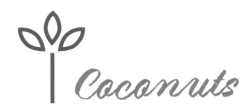

Coconuts

Coconuts are the stone of a drupe (fruit) that grows on large tree-like palms on coastal areas of the tropics (they also grow on plantations inland). The largest of the nuts, they are thought to have originated in tropical Asia and have been used as a food since prehistoric times. Today, they are mainly cultivated in the Philippines, India, Indonesia, Sri Lanka, Mexico, Malaysia and Papua New Guinea, where they are harvested by hand using hooked knives mounted on long bamboo poles to remove them from the trees, or left to fall to the ground. Young 'green' coconuts are harvested in their countries of origin for their juice, and mature coconuts for their juice and their flesh. Coconuts consist of a thick fibrous fruit layer (the husk), within which is a hard, large seed. The seed is enclosed in a hairy shell which has three 'eyes' in one end. The dense white flesh lines the inside of the shell. They are an everyday ingredient in many tropical regions, in South India and Southeast Asia (the South Indian region of Kerala translates as 'the land of the coconuts'). Fresh coconuts feel heavy for their size and when you shake them you should be able to hear the juice sloshing around. They should smell fresh, not rancid. Pierce two of the eyes with a metal skewer and drain out the refreshing, sweet juice before breaking the shell with a hammer or mallet (or chuck it outside against a hard wall or pavement). Fresh coconut flesh has a chewy texture and a mild, nutty and milky flavour that works with both sweet and savoury dishes, and can help to allay the spiciness of chilli-hot dishes. It is covered with a thin brown skin, which can be left on and eaten, or peeled off. The flesh can be frozen, grated or cut into chunks.

NUTRITIONAL BENEFITS
Fresh coconut flesh is rich in fibre, vitamins C and E, B vitamins and minerals including magnesium, potassium, phosphorus, zinc, iron and folic acid. The fresh juice ('water') is a rich source of vitamins and minerals.

SERVING SUGGESTIONS
Eat the coconut flesh in salads or a tropical fruit salad; grate the flesh and use in biscuits, cakes and pastries; make a South Indian chutney with freshly grated coconut, tamarind, mustard seeds and chilli; grate fresh coconut and blitz it with toasted spices and water to make a paste, then add to cooked black beans or green beans and simmer with a little water to make a curry; stir freshly grated and toasted coconut through cooked rice; make a coconut and red lentil dhal.

For coconut 'milk' drink, see page 102.

Coconut products

COCONUT MILK

This rich, thick liquid is made by grating the flesh into water, or pouring boiling water over grated coconut, then straining it. It contains less protein and more fat than cow's milk. Thai brands of coconut milk tend to have the best flavour (choose a brand that specifies in the ingredients list that it contains at least 75 per cent coconut).

Serving suggestions: Add coconut milk to a spicy dressing or salsa; use in a Thai vegetable curry (try pairing aubergines with shiitake mushrooms or green beans, along with lemongrass and Thai basil); stir a little coconut milk into blanched greens with chilli and fried garlic; stew bananas in sweetened coconut milk; add coconut milk to a beetroot or sweet potato soup; make rice pudding with coconut milk and cinnamon or cardamom (or half a vanilla pod), and top with passion fruit or grated chocolate; add to a vegan panna cotta and serve with chargrilled pineapple.

COCONUT CREAM

This thick cream is made by using less water in the coconut-milk production process, and tastes similar. It has a higher fat content than coconut milk and adds a richness and creaminess to dishes without significantly watering them down. You can also find that the coconut milk in tins has separated if it's chilled, and the cream sits in a thick layer at the top of the tin. Only add coconut cream to dishes at the end of the cooking time, as it doesn't tolerate being overheated.

Serving suggestions: Whisk chilled coconut cream as a dairy-free alternative to double cream and serve with fruit and aquafaba meringues; use to make creamy vegan desserts and add to richly spiced sauces.

CREAMED COCONUT

Sometimes confused with coconut cream, creamed coconut is a solid, waxy substance sold as a block of compressed flesh that can be reconstituted to make coconut milk, or used as a substitute for desiccated coconut.

Serving suggestions: Grate and add to savoury curry pastes or a carrot and cardamom halwa (sweet Indian dessert); stir through curries (such as a chickpea curry) at the end of cooking, to help thicken them.

DESICCATED COCONUT

Desiccated coconut is made from the white part of the coconut kernel, after the brown skin has been removed. The white flesh is sterilized, pulped, dried and sieved. It has a fresh coconut taste and is used in confectionary and sweet baked goods. It is available sweetened and unsweetened. Desiccated coconut contains twice as much fibre as almonds.

Serving suggestions: Add to savoury or sweet granolas; use in South Indian chutneys; use unsweetened desiccated coconut in a coating for deep-fried tofu; make a Sri Lankan coconut sambol with fresh chilli, shallots, lime, coconut oil and desiccated coconut; sprinkle over warm coconut-milk porridge.

SHAVED/FLAKED COCONUT

Flaked or shaved coconut pieces are larger than desiccated coconut and are available sweetened and unsweetened. Lightly toast to give them a nuttier flavour and bring out their sweetness.

Serving suggestions: Add to muesli or granola; toast in the oven with oil-rubbed kale leaves; toast and sprinkle over desserts, ice cream made with frozen bananas and mangoes, and breakfast dishes.

COCONUT OIL

Coconut oil, widely used as a cooking oil in South India, is extracted by pressing dried coconut meat. It has a melting point similar to that of milk fat (butter) and is high in saturated fat. It is solid white at room temperature and almost tasteless.

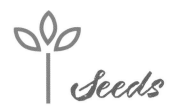

Seeds

Botanically, seeds are the embryo and food supply of new plants and as such are particularly nutritious, packed with vitamins and minerals, iron, healthy oils and protein. They are used to add flavour and texture to dishes. Like nuts, they can be toasted (which enhances their flavour and richness), made into pastes and butters, and can be sprouted or activated (see page 116). Most seeds are valued for their nutritious oils as much as for a food.

POPPY SEEDS

The opium poppy is native to the western Mediterranean and southwestern Asia. Its tiny seeds have been cultivated from the plant's seed pods for thousands of years, both for medicinal purposes and to use in food (it's only the unripe seeds that have narcotic qualities, not the ripe seeds harvested for culinary use). The hard seeds vary from grey-blue (sold as 'black') to light cream. The dark seeds are popular in Central European, Eastern European and Middle Eastern cuisines, used to add crunch and a mildly nutty flavour to savoury and sweet bakes. In India, the ground pale seeds are used as a thickener in savoury dishes and in Japan they are an ingredient in *shichimi togarashi* seasoning mix for noodles and soups. In Jewish cookery they are pounded to a paste, sweetened and used to coat dumplings and bagels. Toasting the seeds strengthens their flavour.

NUTRITIONAL BENEFITS
A good source of minerals (potassium, magnesium and phosphorus).

SERVING SUGGESTIONS
Add poppy seeds to dressings; add a spoonful of seeds to pancake batter; add the black seeds to pale dishes such as a cauliflower salad or a celeriac, cabbage and apple remoulade; scatter over carrots before roasting; use ground and soaked white poppy seeds in coconut-based vegetable curries to act as a thickener; sprout the seeds (see page 95) and add them to salads or use as a garnish; add to a citrus dressing for fruit salad; add the seeds to oatcake dough.

SUNFLOWER SEEDS

These pale brown–grey seeds come from the giant flower heads of the sunflower plant, a North American native, which now grows in temperate climates worldwide. The flower heads contain anything from several hundred to 2,000 seeds. They were used as a food by North American Indians for thousands of years, who extracted the oil from the seeds, and dried or roasted then ground them to use in cakes or soups. The seeds are sold with their stripy black and white or black shell intact, or hulled. They have an oily, slightly sweet taste, which is enhanced when toasted, and are high in protein.

NUTRITIONAL BENEFITS
A rich source of vitamin E, B vitamins, minerals, protein, iron and calcium.

SERVING SUGGESTIONS
Add to bread dough, along with other seeds; toast and sprinkle over a vegetable pilaf; toast with soy sauce and use as a garnish for an Asian salad; add to a nutty granola; sprinkle into stir-fries or over roast butternut squash; make a savoury crumble with oats, sunflower seeds, nuts and breadcrumbs; caramelize in a frying pan with a little sugar and sprinkle over puddings.

PUMPKIN SEEDS

The dark green seeds of large squash varieties native to the Americas. The seeds are most often sold with their pale oval shells (husks) removed. The teardrop-shaped seeds have a delicately nutty flavour and chewy texture and can be eaten raw or cooked. In South America they are known as *pipián* and are roasted and ground to use as a thickener in savoury sauces (*mole*) for tacos, burritos or enchiladas. Pumpkin seeds are used as a garnish, and a snack. They are rich in healthy oils, contain more iron than any other seed and more protein than peanuts. To enhance their nuttiness, roast before using. When fresh pumpkins are in season, remove the seeds and roast them in their hulls.

NUTRITIONAL BENEFITS

A rich source of protein, iron, zinc, potassium, vitamins A and E, B vitamins and phosphorus.

SERVING SUGGESTIONS

Add the seeds to bread dough; scatter toasted seeds over a pumpkin and sage risotto; make pumpkin seed pesto; make pumpkin seed butter (using the same technique as nut butters – see page 162); toast, add maple syrup then leave to cool before chopping and sprinkling over desserts; add toasted seeds to date, cocoa and hazelnut energy balls; toast the seeds and sprinkle over a fennel, quinoa and orange salad.

LINSEEDS

Linseeds (also called flaxseeds) come from the flax plant, which is native to India. It is cultivated in temperate and tropical regions for its fibre (used to make linen) and its glossy seed (used primarily to make oil, but also for the seed). Linseeds are particularly rich in healthy omega-3 fats and high in fibre, and have a mild ,nutty flavour. The seeds are often reddish-brown, but can also be dark yellow, depending on the variety, and are sold whole or milled (ground). They need to be ground in order to make their nutrients accessible and are best used raw,

Other seeds

HEMP SEEDS: Native to Central Asia and first cultivated in China, hemp seeds are a rich source of healthy oils, proteins, minerals and vitamin E. They can be roasted or eaten raw, and used in both sweet and savoury dishes. Hemp seeds are used to make a type of tofu, using a similar production process, which can be baked or crumbled into savoury dishes. Combine the mildly nutty seeds with herb and spice rubs to use as a seasoning, or add to smoothies.

CHIA SEEDS: These mottled grey seeds, native to Mexico and Guatemala and appreciated in these regions since Mayan times, have a distinctive crunchy texture and mild flavour, and are a rich source of healthy oils and an excellent source of vitamin E and minerals. They are sold milled or whole. Soak them until they swell, then add to smoothies, porridge, granola or bread. They develop a gelatinous texture when soaked, so make a good alternative to eggs in vegan puddings.

How to activate nuts, grains and seeds

This is the first step of sprouting (see page 95). It stimulates germination, converts proteins into easily digestible amino acids, is a faster way to increase the bioavailability of nutrients than sprouting and hydrates the nut/grain/seed.

- Rinse seeds, grains or nuts then place in a bowl and cover with salted water (2 teaspoons salt for 2 cups of seeds/grains/nuts).

- Soak for 7–12 hours at room temperature, covered with a clean cloth, then strain and use. The soaking time depends on the size of the ingredient you are soaking.

- At this stage, they're ready for making milks (see page 102)

Nuts need to be dehydrated in a very low oven after being soaked, until they are dry, but seeds and legumes do not require this.

Nuts and seeds that take well to being activated include hulled pumpkin seeds, sunflower seeds and almonds (use raw nuts and seeds, not roasted).

not cooked. Linseed oil is a good alternative to fish oil as a dietary supplement (avoid heating the oil, which can destroy some of its beneficial nutrients). Linseeds can also be sprouted (see page 95).

NUTRITIONAL BENEFITS
A good source of fibre, magnesium, omega-3 fatty acids and zinc.

SERVING SUGGESTIONS
Add ground seeds to bread dough or make German *leinsamenbrot* (linseed bread); sprinkle ground linseeds over salads; make linseed crackers; soak the seeds in water overnight, then add to smoothies, porridge or granola; combine ground seeds with breadcrumbs to make a crunchy coating for deep-fried tofu or other vegetables of your choosing.

SESAME SEEDS

These are one of the most ancient oilseed crops. Native to India, sesame made its way through the Asian subcontinent and Anatolia over thousands of years, reaching China by the second century BCE – China is now the world's largest consumer of the seed. Sesame seeds are available in a wide variety of colours, but black and white are the most common. The white seeds are milder than the dark, but both have a delicate taste and add texture and nuttiness to sweet and savoury dishes. In China, both are used (the black seeds are ground to make a sweet paste for confectionary and puddings); in India the white sesame seed is preferred, as a spice and in sweet dishes; in Japan, unhulled sesame seeds are ground with salt to make a condiment called *gomashio*, and the seeds are sprinkled over rice or noodles; and in the Middle East, they are eaten toasted or raw, used in baking, or made into tahini (see opposite). Toasting them makes them aromatic and nutty.

NUTRITIONAL BENEFITS
A good source of protein and calcium, vitamin B_3 and niacin. Just 25g (1oz) provides nearly half the recommended RDA of iron.

Grind with sea salt to make a condiment for savoury dishes; scatter toasted seeds over fried apple or banana fritters; add black sesame seeds to citrus cake batters; sprinkle seeds over baked figs; add to a fruit crumble mixture; add white seeds to Chinese 'smashed' cucumbers, along with toasted sesame oil; sprinkle seeds into an apple and celeriac salad, or over a cool noodle and vegetable salad with a chilli-spiked dressing; scatter over grilled miso aubergine or baba ganoush; combine tahini, miso, lemon juice, sesame oil and sesame seeds to make a dressing for steamed broccoli; make sesame-seed dukkah and sprinkle over roast squash or sweet potato; add seeds to a dipping sauce for Vietnamese vegetarian spring rolls; sprinkle toasted seeds over an Asian-style mango, watercress and herb salad; roll falafel in raw sesame seeds before baking or frying; make sesame brittle with maple syrup and white sesame seeds.

Tahini

This nutritious, oily paste made from hulled sesame seeds is synonymous with the vast and varied cuisines of the Middle East, where it is often loosened with cold water and lemon juice (and sometimes garlic) to drizzle over savoury dishes and serve as a dip with mezze, or combined with chickpeas to make hummus. Tahini is also a key component of sweet, crumbly halva. It is rich in protein and there are two types: light and dark – the light is made with hulled seeds and is considered finer in taste and texture than the dark, nutty tahini which includes the hulls. Chinese and Japanese sesame pastes are made from roasted unhulled sesame seeds.

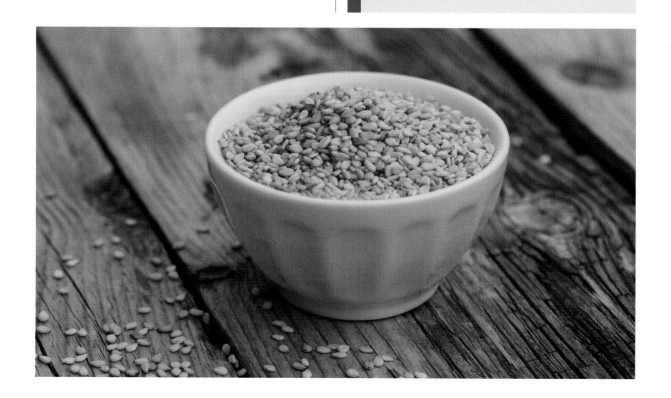

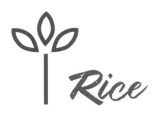

Rice

The Asian plant that produces rice was introduced by the Arabs to Europe in the tenth century where it was first cultivated in Spain, then Italy, reaching the Americas by the sixteenth and seventeenth centuries. Thousands of varieties are cultivated on every continent and it is a staple, starch-rich food for at least half the world's population. There are two key types – long-grain rice and short-grain rice – and most rice is refined: milled to remove the bran and most of the germ, then 'polished'. Rice is available as pre-cooked and quick-cook rice; itis also used to make flour, milk and noodles, and fermented to make vinegars, wine and sake.

LONG-GRAIN WHITE RICE

This versatile rice has an elongated, slender shape and a subtle, mildly sweet flavour. Its texture is firmer than basmati rice. It is pearled or 'polished' rice that has been refined by having the fibrous bran and germ layers removed. This process removes most of the nutrients, though many producers enrich them to improve their nutritional profiles. The grains, when cooked properly, remain distinct. Popular in China, India and North America. Rinse before using.

NUTRITIONAL BENEFITS
A source of protein (and most white rice is enriched with nutrients, including iron and B vitamins, during processing).

SERVING SUGGESTIONS
Stir cooked, peeled broad beans and chopped dill through cooked rice; cook rice with quinoa or other grains to boost its nutritional content; make a vegan *nasi goreng* with cooked rice, onions, garlic, carrots, shredded greens, soy sauce, lime juice and chilli sauce; make a vegan version of the Creole classic, jambalaya, with long-grain rice, Cajun spices, red peppers, tomatoes and an onion; make Caribbean rice and peas.

BROWN RICE

Wholegrain rice contains the bran, germ and endosperm of the grain and is more nutritious than white rice. It is used more widely in the West than in countries such as Japan and China where rice is a staple ingredient. When cooked, it has a chewy texture and a rich aroma, though it can take two to three times longer than white rice to become tender. Brown rice is available as long-, medium- or short-grain rice and fragrant rice. Rinse well and soak before cooking to rid the rice of dust and shorten the cooking time.

NUTRITIONAL BENEFITS
A good source of protein, fibre, calcium and B vitamins.

SERVING SUGGESTIONS
Add cooked brown rice to a Korean bibimbap rice bowl with pickled and/or sautéed vegetables, tofu and Korean spices; stir-fry cooked brown rice with vegetables and ginger; make kheer (Indian spiced rice pudding) with almond milk and soaked brown rice; make rice burgers; use organic rice to make *horchata*, a nutritious cold drink made by blitzing soaked rice with almond milk, vanilla, cinnamon and maple syrup.

BASMATI RICE

A long-grain aromatic white or brown rice grown in the foothills of the Himalayas, the Punjab regions of India and Pakistan and used in many south Asian and Middle Eastern cuisines, primarily in savoury dishes. The slender grains have a delicate nut-like, fruity flavour and remain separate when cooked (but can become claggy if overcooked). In most cases the grains are pearled or 'polished' and have their fibrous bran and germ layers removed. Premium varieties are often aged to improve their flavour. Soaking the rice before cooking (30 minutes is sufficient) shortens the cooking time, retaining more of its aromatic qualities.

NUTRITIONAL BENEFITS
A source of protein (most white rice is enriched with nutrients, including iron and B vitamins, during processing).

SERVING SUGGESTIONS
Cook rice in saffron-infused water and scatter with toasted pine nuts; make a vegetable biryani and scatter with nigella seeds; make a broad bean or chickpea and lemon pilaf; make *khichidi*, an Indian rice and lentil dish, with yellow or red split lentils, cinnamon and turmeric; add cooked rice to a stir-fry of spring vegetables and ginger and season with soy sauce and nutritional yeast; add cooked rice to Mexican black beans cooked with tomato and paprika, and use to fill a burrito.

RISOTTO RICE

The creamy-textured Italian dish of risotto is made with plump medium- to long-grain rice cultivated specifically for the dish. Of the many varieties of risotto rice, Arborio and Carnaroli are the most common. Like basmati rice and long-grain white rice, the grains are pearled or 'polished' and white. Stirring the rice during cooking, while gradually adding hot liquid (often a light stock, known as 'brodo' in Italy), coaxes starch from the outer layers of the grains, which thickens the risotto and gives it a creamy, rich consistency. The rice is cooked when it is tender but still has a chalky – but not crunchy – 'bite' in the centre. Toasting the rice in oil and sautéed onion or shallot briefly before you add the liquid (the first liquid added is often wine) helps stop the rice from getting mushy. Carnaroli rice remains a little firmer than other risotto rice varieties, so is less easy to overcook. Don't rinse the rice before using. Risotto rice can also be used to make rice pudding.

NUTRITIONAL BENEFITS
A source of protein (most white rice is enriched with nutrients, including iron and B vitamins, during processing).

SERVING SUGGESTIONS
Make *risi e bisi*, a Venetian rice soup of risotto rice with young cooked peas; make a broad bean risotto (add bean pods to the stock if you have them), nettle or mushroom risotto (using the soaking liquid from dried mushrooms in the stock, as well as fresh mushrooms); stuff courgette flowers with leftover risotto, then fry in oil; stir ribbons of lettuce through a cooked plain risotto just before serving.

PAELLA RICE

Another pearled or 'polished' rice, this short- to medium-grain rice is grown in Spain for making the traditional Valencian dish, paella. 'Paella' is the name of the flat pan with a circular base in which the dish is cooked, and the Spanish region from where it originates. Paella rice with DO (Denomination of Origin) certification, such as Calasparra and Valencia, indicates a high-quality grain. Bomba is the most widely used. Don't rinse the rice before cooking, as the starch is key to the dish's texture. Traditionally, the paella is shaken, not stirred, so that the rice on the bottom of the pan forms a sought-after and delicious crust.

NUTRITIONAL BENEFITS
A source of protein (most white rice is enriched with nutrients, including iron and B vitamins, during processing).

SERVING SUGGESTIONS
Make a vegetable paella with green beans, red peppers, tomatoes, olive oil, paprika and saffron; add smoked tofu or fried mushrooms to a green bean paella; make paella with broad beans and peas; use paella rice instead of pudding rice to make a sweet rice pudding, cooking the grains in almond milk and sprinkling ground almonds on top to serve, and a little maple syrup or sugar.

SUSHI RICE

Many Japanese short-grain white rice varieties that are used to make sushi and other Japanese dishes are sold as 'sushi rice': they all share a characteristic stickiness when cooked, which enable them to be moulded and cling together well enough to be easily picked up with chopsticks. Japanese rice is available in wholegrain brown form and white hulled form and is a staple in Japan, where almost no meal is complete without a bowl of it. To rinse the rice, put it in a pan, fill the pan with water, swish the rice around with your hand for a few minutes, then drain and repeat the process with fresh water, until the water is clear. Cook until tender, drain, cover and leave to steam, then fluff up (brown rice is not as sticky as white and takes longer to cook).

NUTRITIONAL BENEFITS
A source of protein (most white rice is enriched with nutrients, including iron and B vitamins, during processing).

SERVING SUGGESTIONS
Make vegetable *makizushi* (sushi rolls) with cooked sushi rice and nori sheets, filling them with avocado and pickled ginger or grated carrot; make rice pudding with coconut milk and sushi rice; serve plain, cooked sushi rice with miso soup and steamed greens; sprinkle cooked brown sushi rice with a rice vinegar dressing, then serve in a bowl with soya beans, avocado, nori and pickled ginger, radish or daikon and cucumber ribbons; add cooked brown sushi rice to a stir-fry; serve cooked sushi rice with fried firm tofu and soy-fried shiitake mushrooms.

WILD RICE

Wild rice is the seed of a marsh grass that grows in shallow water, rather than a grain. It is the only cereal grain from North America to have become important as a human food and – contrary to its name – is largely commercially cultivated. After harvesting, the rice is matured, dried over heat, then threshed to remove the husk. Wild rice is a whole grain with a complex, nutty and tea-like flavour and a firm, chewy texture when cooked. The shiny dark grains take longer to cook than most grains, splitting when cooked.

NUTRITIONAL BENEFITS
High in protein, B vitamins and a good source of fibre.

SERVING SUGGESTIONS
Mix with cooked grains in a salad while the rice is still warm, so it soaks up more of the dressing; combine with cooked quinoa, grilled asparagus and fried mushrooms; combine cooked wild rice with ripe mangoes, coriander and a citrus dressing, and serve in lettuce cups; make a wild rice pilaf with preserved lemons and pistachios.

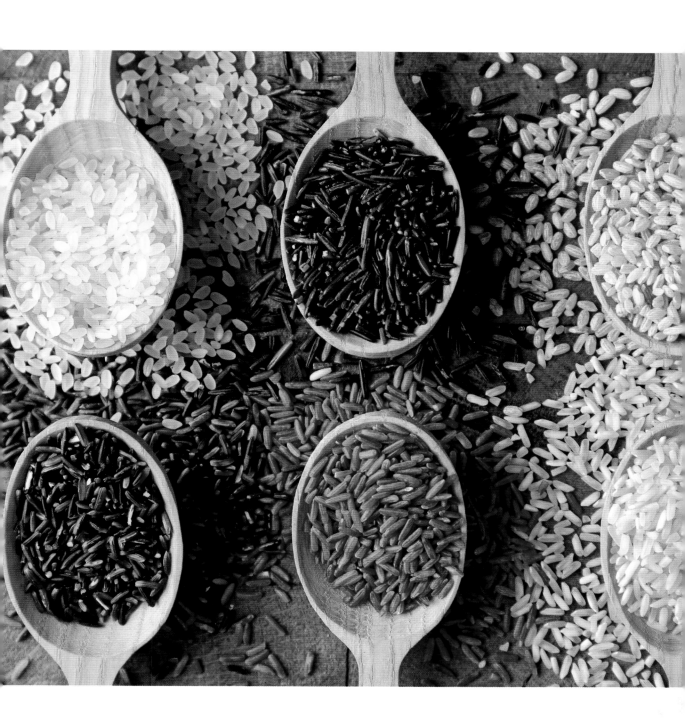

Pasta

Pasta is one of the most popular, simple and satisfying foods in the world. The word 'pasta' means 'paste' or 'dough' in Italian, and at its most basic, the dough is made with just flour and water.

There are many ways to categorize pasta, but commonly, in Italy, its many forms fall into one of two groups: flour-and-water pastas, and the richer egg-and-flour pastas. Flour-and-water pastas are usually factory-made with durum wheat semolina (see page 128), then dried; egg pasta is usually sold fresh or handmade and is made with soft wheat flour, but can also be factory-made.

In factories, pasta shapes are made by extruding the dough through perforated dies then drying the shapes. Superior factory-made pasta is made using traditional bronze dies rather than Teflon dies, which gives the pasta a slightly rougher surface (sauces cling better to these pastas).

In Italy, pasta is a staple food that's usually served at the start of a meal, but it is also made and eaten the world over. Venezuela is the world's second largest consumer after Italy; in China, flour-and-water dough is used to make noodles; and in the Middle East, Greece, Spain and Mexico, vermicelli appears in both sweet and savoury dishes. Spaghetti – that most famous of pastas – accounts for over half of the world's pasta consumption.

Pasta is available fresh or dry, wholewheat or white, flavoured, and dyed (often with the juice of spinach or beetroot, or tomato paste), and in wheat-free forms, made with ingredients such as rice, quinoa, black beans, edamame beans or chestnut flour.

SAUCES, PESTOS AND BAKES

Pasta's neutral taste makes it an ideal vehicle for other flavours. The pasta suggestions here aren't intended to be prescriptive – feel free to choose your favourite pasta-and-sauce combination.

– **Chickpea sauce:** Sauté onion and garlic with some chopped rosemary, add tinned or cooked chickpeas and a little vegetable stock, and simmer until soft. Blitz half the sauce, leave half the chickpeas whole. Serve with orecchiette, farfalle or vermicelli.

tip

Check packets to make sure the pasta you are buying is made without eggs. Italian dry pasta made with eggs will have 'all'uovo' on the packet wording.

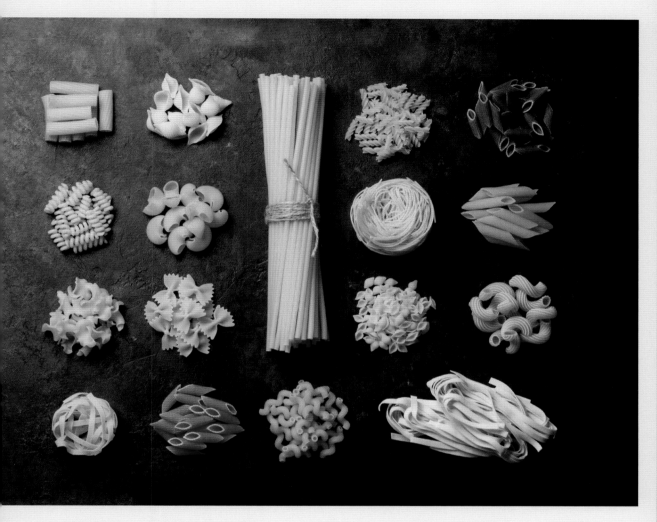

- **Meatless meatballs and tomato sauce:** Sauté finely chopped mushrooms and garlic in oil, then add chopped thyme, cooked green or puy lentils and sun-dried tomato paste. Blitz to combine, then roll into balls, adding breadcrumbs to help the mixture hold together, if necessary. Fry until browned. Make a simple tomato sauce with onion, olive oil and tinned tomatoes, then add the meatballs. Serve with tagliatelle, fettuccine or orzo.

- **Walnut sauce:** Crush garlic, walnuts and parsley using a pestle and mortar with some vegan-milk-soaked breadcrumbs, then gradually stir in olive oil. Coat the pasta in the sauce. Serve with spaghetti or linguine.

- **Lasagne:** Make a vegan béchamel and lentil ragu, layer with quick-cook or part-cooked lasagne and bake, or use slices of aubergine, spicy tomato sauce and vegan 'mozzarella'.

- **Brussels sprout, sage and pine nut sauce:** Sauté shredded Brussels sprouts and garlic in oil, add pine nuts and lemon zest and cook until the nuts are toasted. Serve with tagliatelle or tagliolini.

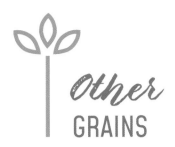

Other GRAINS

Wheat and corn are the most common food grains, but there are many others that offer a wide variety of flavours, nutritional qualities and textures, including the pseudo-grains amaranth, buckwheat and quinoa, which are used in a similar way so are featured here. These important sources of carbohydrate are available ground and processed, but grains are at their most nutritious in their whole form. Most grains, unless you buy them toasted, benefit from an initial dry-toasting in the pan before they are cooked, to give them greater depth of flavour.

CORNMEAL

This milled, ground corn (maize), native to the Americas, is available in myriad guises: coarse, medium or fine in texture, and in shades from white and gold through to blue. It is sometimes sold as 'polenta', the name of the Italian dish of cooked cornmeal, or 'grits' in the USA, and is a staple food crop in corn-growing regions. Some of the many dishes made with this versatile grain include American cornbread, north Italian polenta, Jamaican deep-fried dumplings, Italian cakes and Romanian porridge. It has a bland, mildly sweet flavour and is an ideal, soft-textured base for more assertive ingredients and creamy, rich dishes. Cornmeal is also used in baking. To make polenta on the hob, use five times the volume of salted water (or a mixture of vegan milk and water) to coarse yellow or white cornmeal. Bring the water to the boil, remove the pan from the heat and pour in the cornmeal, whisking continuously. Return to a low heat and cook following the packet instructions (it can take anything from 5 minutes to 45 minutes), stirring frequently.

NUTRITIONAL BENEFITS
A good source of fibre, zinc, iron, niacin and protein.

SERVING SUGGESTIONS
Slice cool and firm polenta, then grill or fry; make an olive oil, cornmeal and rosemary cake or cornmeal, orange and almond cake; bake cornmeal in the oven with vegetable stock, herbs and spices; fry wedges of cooked polenta and serve with home-made baked beans; use cornmeal to crumb-coat sticks of aubergine or courgette before frying; use coarse cornmeal to make a vegan cornbread; make polenta and serve as a bed for fried mushrooms.

POPCORN

This popular snack food comes from a small variety of corn with a tough hull and endosperm that's grown specifically cultivated for the purpose. For thousands of years, these kernels have been popped. Records show that the Aztecs, Incas and North American tribes of the New Mexico were eating popcorn over 5,000 years ago. These days it remains a beloved snack. When heated in a covered pan (with oil or no oil), the kernel swells, forms steam and explodes with a popping sound, turning the kernel inside out in the process, so that the starchy part is outside the shell. This stiffens a little as it cools, forming the light and crisp snack that so many of us associate with those enormous cinema tubs. It is often salted or sweetened (or both).

NUTRITIONAL BENEFITS
A good source of fibre, protein and manganese.

SERVING SUGGESTIONS
To make popcorn, toast a small quantity of dried corn kernels with a little oil in a large, heavy-based lidded saucepan (with the lid slightly ajar, so steam can escape) and place over a high heat, shaking frequently, until they all pop – you'll know it's ready when 2–3 seconds elapse between 'pops'; toss popped corn with melted chocolate and a mixture of cocoa powder and icing sugar; toss in melted vegan butter, cinnamon and maple syrup; toss in a mixture of ground nutritional yeast, sugar and chilli, or a herbed salt.

CRACKED WHEAT

Wheat is native to Southwest Asia and the largest and most important grain crop. Cracked wheat is made from raw durum wheat berries (whole wheat grains with the husks removed) that are crushed or roughly broken. They retain all the nutrients of the whole wheat grain and can be used as an alternative to rice and other grains and in bread-making. Cracked wheat is often confused with bulgur wheat, which is a partially cooked wheat berry. When cooked, it has a slightly sticky feel and a nuttiness and palatable crunchiness. Freekeh, a popular grain in the Middle East, is the young ('green') wheat which has been roasted in the husk, hulled and sold whole or cracked (cracked freekeh cooks more quickly). It has a smoky, nutty flavour and can be cooked like rice or barley.

NUTRITIONAL BENEFITS
A good source of B vitamins, vitamins A and E, fibre and protein.

SERVING SUGGESTIONS
Serve cooked cracked wheat in a herb-packed salad alongside grilled vegetables; cook cracked freekeh in a vegetable stew; add cracked wheat and seeds to bread dough before baking; use cracked wheat or freekeh to make a pilaf; add cracked wheat to a spicy vegan chilli.

BULGUR WHEAT

This part-cooked, cracked durum wheat, together with an abundance of fresh herbs, is the key ingredient in the Middle Eastern salad, tabbouleh, and features frequently in Middle Eastern and North African cuisines. It has been made for centuries by partially cooking the whole grains, drying them, then moistening them to toughen the outer bran, before milling to remove the bran and germ and grinding to form either coarse or fine bulgur. Fibre-rich bulgur wheat is nutritious, keeps well and cooks quickly: it often just needs to be soaked in just-boiled water or stock for 15–30 minutes to become light, fluffy and nutty.

tip

Coarse bulgur can be cooked in a similar style to rice and couscous, fine bulgur is usually used to make falafel.

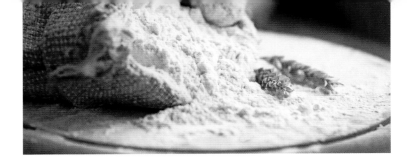

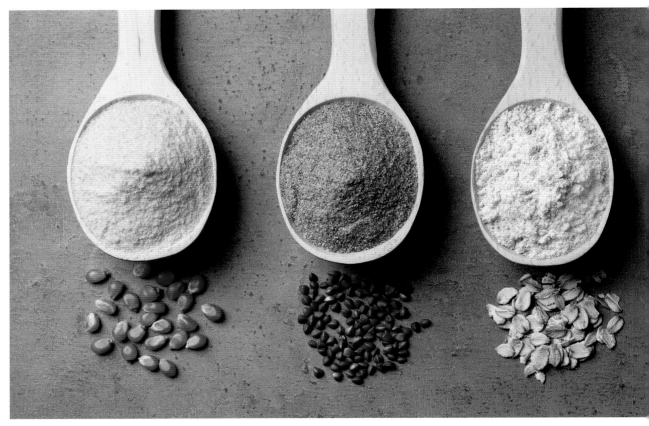

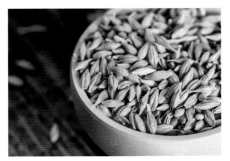

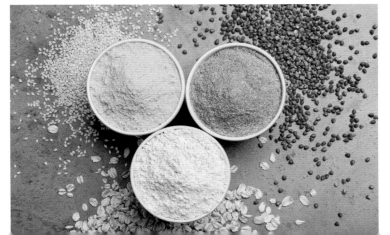

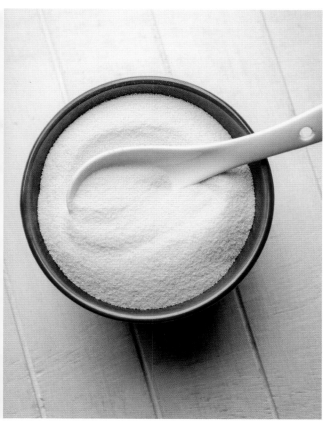

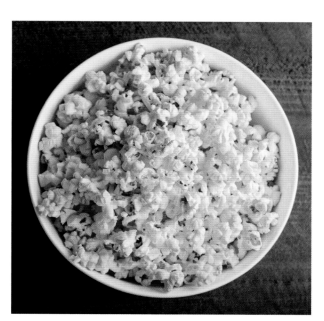

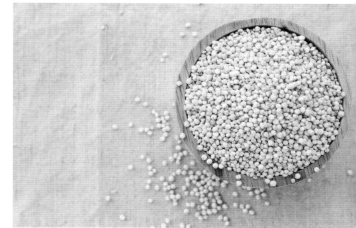

NUTRITIONAL BENEFITS

A good source of manganese, magnesium, protein and iron.

SERVING SUGGESTIONS

Make a tabbouleh-style salad with cooked bulgur wheat, chopped soft herbs, tomatoes and cucumber, and toss with an olive oil and lemon juice dressing; make a bulgur wheat pilaf and sprinkle with dried barberries and chopped pistachios; cook coarse bulgur wheat in stock, with allspice and sautéed shallots, and scatter with sumac; make vegetarian kibbeh with roast squash, cooked bulgur wheat and chickpeas.

SEMOLINA

Semolina is made from the central kernel of milled durum wheat or hard wheat. It is similar in appearance to cornmeal and has a sand-like granular texture, with varying degrees of coarseness. It appears in both savoury and sweet dishes, from Indian, Scandinavian and Middle Eastern puddings to Italian pasta and gnocchi, and in bread- and cake-baking. Semolina has a higher protein and gluten content than soft wheat flour. In southern Italy, semolina is often used alone or blended with finer 00-grade wheat flour and water in pasta-making (in the north of Italy, egg pasta is more common). Semolina is mostly amber in colour, but can also be white.

NUTRITIONAL BENEFITS

A good source of fibre and vitamin E.

SERVING SUGGESTIONS

Toss par-boiled potatoes in seasoned semolina before roasting, to give them extra crunch; to make a soothing pudding, whisk semolina into a pan of simmering vegan milk and cook for about 5 minutes, then stir in sugar to taste, and a little almond extract; make a flatbread dough or pizza base using a 50/50 blend of white flour and semolina; cook it with vegan milk, like polenta, to make a creamy side dish; make pasta (see page 122).

COUSCOUS

Couscous is often mistaken for a grain, when in fact, it is made of durum wheat semolina dough, which is rubbed to form tiny balls. It hails from North Africa, where it is a staple, sustaining food, served with stews and tagines, and in salads. Traditionally, it is cooked in a lengthy process that requires repeatedly steaming it in a muslin-lined steamer or *couscousiere* (designed specifically for the job), but conveniently, most couscous is available pre-cooked and only requires brief rehydrating in hot water or stock until it swells. Couscous comes in several sizes, from giant (also called 'pearl' couscous) to fine-grained, and wholewheat couscous is particularly nutritious. Fregola is a Sardinian speciality, a bead-shaped pasta traditionally made using the same technique as couscous. A large Palestinian couscous-style product, known as *maftoul*, is made from sun-dried bulgur wheat and can be cooked like rice.

NUTRITIONAL BENEFITS

A good source of fibre and vitamin E.

SERVING SUGGESTIONS

Combine cooked couscous with raisins, pine nuts and chopped preserved lemon; serve warm couscous with a spiced vegetable stew, and scatter with pomegranate seeds; add cooked fregola to a salad of roasted tomatoes and basil; toss cooked couscous with chickpeas, drizzle with a citrus dressing and scatter with toasted almonds and caramelized onions; combine cooked fregola or maftoul with mung beans or broad beans and serve with roasted vegetables.

tip

Toast couscous in a dry pan
before rehydrating it to give it
an appealing nuttiness.

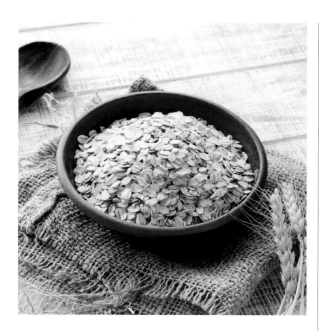

OATS

Likely native to southwestern Asia, oats have been an important, fibre-rich staple in Northern European human and animal diets for millennia, though their use as a human food took time to take hold, no thanks to the ancient Romans and Greeks who considered it a coarse product fit for only cattle. Oats have a sweet flavour and creamy texture when cooked, and contain more protein than most grains. Most oats are cultivated in cool climates of the northern hemisphere and are roasted and processed to varying degrees to make products primarily used in slow-cooked savoury dishes, baking and in porridge: these range from groats – whole hulled oats – to fine oatmeal and oatbran (the outer casing of the seed and fruit of the oat kernel).

NUTRITIONAL BENEFITS
A good source of B vitamins, vitamin E, calcium, zinc, iron, magnesium, phosphorus, potassium, fibre and protein.

SERVING SUGGESTIONS
Add rolled oats to smoothies; add rolled oats to a mixed-grain bread dough; add rolled or jumbo oats to a nutty crumble mixture or granola; toast rolled oats with flaxseeds, then add vegan milk, warm spices and syrup and simmer until cooked to make porridge; make oatmeal biscuits or crispbreads, using a mixture of fine and coarse oatmeal; add oats to vegan flapjacks; make bircher muesli with rolled or jumbo oats, vegan milk of choice and water, then serve with fruit; use coarse oatmeal or groats instead of barley in a vegetable stew; use medium oatmeal in a crumb coating for vegetables before frying.

BARLEY

Barley is native to the fertile grasslands of southwestern Asia, from where it migrated to Europe, North Africa and Asia. It is one of the oldest known cultivated grains and was a common foodstuff until the Middle Ages, particularly as a flour, but it now occupies a peripheral place in the world of edible grains (much of the world's crop is used in brewing and distilling, or to make miso, see page 99). It deserves greater attention as an ingredient, however, as it is a sweet, fibre-rich grain with a lovely nuttiness. Wholegrain, hulled 'pot' barley is brown and firm-textured when cooked, and pearl barley is the softer, polished grain, with both the hull and bran removed. Pearl barley cooks more quickly than pot barley, and has a mild, sweet flavour and chewy texture but is less nutritious: semi-pearled barley is a good middle-ground, as it still retains some of the grain's bran.

NUTRITIONAL BENEFITS
A good source of B vitamins, vitamin E, calcium, copper, iodine, iron, magnesium, selenium, potassium and fibre.

SERVING SUGGESTIONS
Use pearl barley instead of risotto rice to make a mushroom risotto; make a millet and barley pilaf; make barley water, a traditional rejuvenating beverage, by simmering pearl barley in water for 1 hour, then straining and sweetening the water with maple syrup and lemon or orange juice to taste – leave to cool then chill; cook pearl barley gently in water or vegan milk, then add raisins and apples or fruit compote and sweeten to taste; add cooked pot or pearl barley to a mushroom or celeriac soup; add cooked pot barley to a vegetable stew.

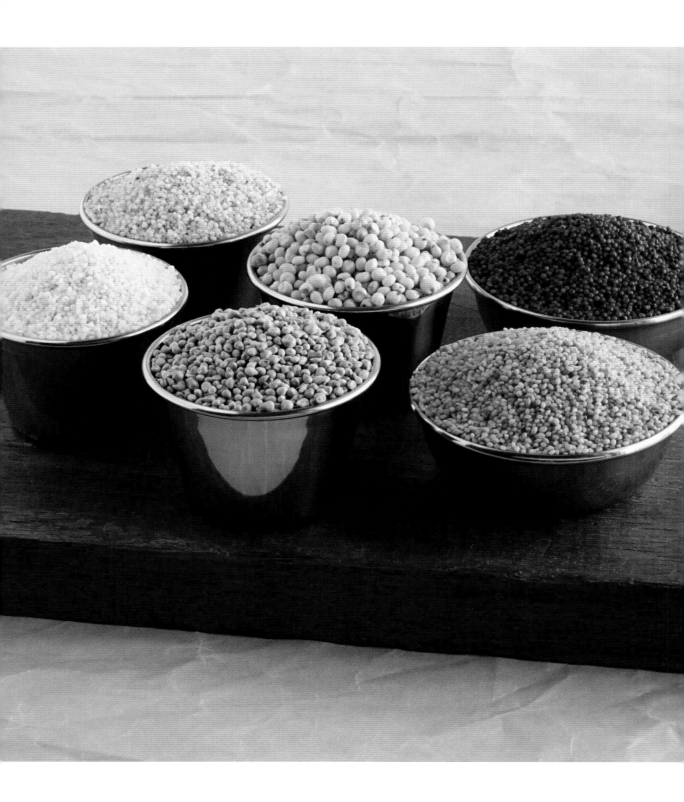

QUINOA

Quinoa is native to South America and was a key source of food for the ancient Andeans and Incans (the Incans called it 'the mother of all grains'). This pseudo-cereal grain (it is a seed rather than a grass) is cultivated in the US, Bolivia, Peru, China and the UK and has impressive health credentials, being high in fibre and an excellent source of protein. The small, pearlescent, bead-shaped spheres come in a variety of shades, from white and gold to black, red or orange, and have a springy texture and a grassy, slightly astringent flavour.

The seeds are processed to make flaked quinoa (steamed, rolled and dried seeds), whole quinoa and quinoa flour. When cooked, quinoa seeds swell to about four times their original size and become almost translucent. Rinse quinoa well under cold running water, until the water runs clear, to reduce bitterness, then cook it like rice. Measure double the volume of water or stock to quinoa. Toast it in oil, then add the water or stock, bring to the boil, reduce the heat, cover and cook for 10–15 minutes. Rest for 5 minutes, covered, then fluff with a fork.

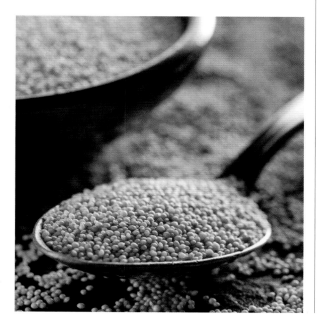

NUTRITIONAL BENEFITS
A good source of calcium, phosphorus and iron, and vitamin E.

SERVING SUGGESTIONS
Use quinoa instead of bulgur wheat to make tabbouleh; swap rice for quinoa in a pilaf; make porridge with quinoa flakes; add cooked quinoa to a vegetable stew; stir cooked quinoa through grilled courgettes and onion, and dress with olive oil and lemon juice (top with toasted nuts, if you like); add cooked quinoa to a vegetable wrap; mix cooked quinoa with crushed black beans, sautéed onion and spices to make burgers.

SPELT

Spelt is one of the most ancient varieties of cultivated wheat. Regions where it is grown include Central and Eastern Europe, and it is particularly appreciated in Germany, for brewing as well as eating. The low yields of spelt crops compared to common wheat crops, and the toughness of their husks, have led to it playing a marginal role in European cuisines, however it is a richer source of protein, vitamins and minerals than regular wheat, contains less gluten, and has a reputation for being easier to digest than wheat flour. Spelt is available as a whole (hulled) grain, a white, polished (pearled) grain, and a flour. In Central Europe the under-ripe grain is often gently roasted and ground to use in soups, and in Germany (where it is known as dinkel wheat) it is used in baking. The grains have a complex, nutty, sweet flavour when cooked.

NUTRITIONAL BENEFITS
A good source of protein, minerals, iron, zinc and B vitamins.

SERVING SUGGESTIONS
Swap risotto rice for pearled spelt when making a risotto; make bread or cookies with spelt flour; team cooked spelt with roasted root vegetables; add pearled spelt to a mushroom soup; toss cooked spelt through a warm broccoli salad with a miso dressing.

MILLET

Various kinds of millets, native to Africa and Asia, are grown for their small, edible grains, for both human and animal consumption. It has been an important staple food in many hot, dry countries for thousands of years. In its native growing regions, millet is used in bread-making, and cooked with milk, water or stock to serve served alongside savoury dishes or as a creamy porridge. The round, golden grains are highly nutritious, particularly rich in iron and protein, and are available hulled, in whole, cracked and puffed form, and as flakes and flour. Millet has a slightly nutty, mild flavour. To emphasise this nuttiness, toast the grains briefly before using. The grains cook and swell to many times their original size when cooked, so use sparingly: rinse and cook with three times the volume of water to millet for 10–12 minutes in boiling water or stock, then leave to rest for a few minutes before fluffing with a fork. Or, cook it for longer, with more liquid, until it becomes thick and smooth, like polenta. It works well in place of rice, couscous or quinoa in savoury dishes.

NUTRITIONAL BENEFITS
A good source of iron, magnesium, phosphorus, zinc, calcium, B vitamins, fibre and protein.

SERVING SUGGESTIONS
Add cooked whole millet to vegetable burger mixtures; substitute for rice and serve with a vegetable curry; cook whole millet with coconut milk to make porridge; add millet flakes to bread dough, biscuits or muesli; add cooked whole millet to a warm vegetable salad; make a millet pilaf.

BUCKWHEAT

Despite its name, buckwheat is neither a wheat nor a grain – it is a small brown triangular seed. Central Asia is thought to be the plant's native region, and it reached Europe in the Middle Ages, where it was cultivated as a minor grain crop. Buckwheat is milled to make a flour, and sold whole and hulled as toasted or untoasted

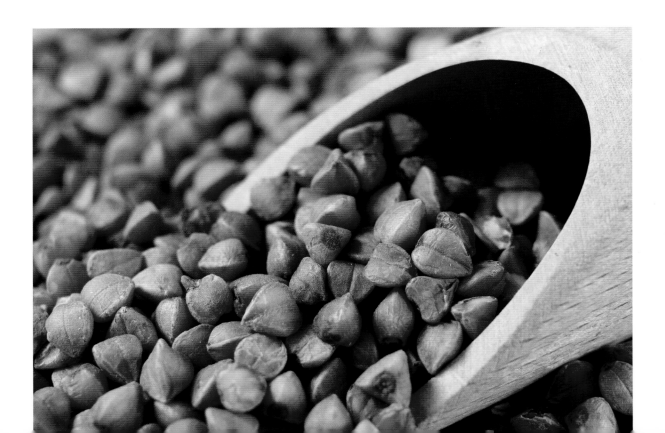

raw groats. The flour is used to make soba noodles, pasta, pancakes and bread (mixed with other flours, as buckwheat contains no gluten). Toasted groats are called *kasha* and are typically used to make a porridge of the same name in Russia and parts of Eastern Europe. Of all the pseudo-grains and grains in this section, buckwheat has the strongest flavour; an earthy taste that's almost astringent. It therefore lends itself best to hearty, savoury dishes. It is a useful alternative to wheat for those with intolerances or allergies.

NUTRITIONAL BENEFITS
A good source of vitamin A, B vitamins, iron, protein, calcium and selenium.

SERVING SUGGESTIONS
Make buckwheat pancakes with buckwheat flour, or buckwheat porridge for kasha, and top with sautéed mushrooms; add a palmful of kasha or raw buckwheat to risotto rice before cooking; mix whole raw buckwheat into granola mixtures before baking; mix cooked buckwheat into a roasted squash salad with herbs and a creamy tahini dressing.

AMARANTH

Native to Mexico and Central and South America, this tiny seed resembles quinoa and is another pseudo-grain that was eaten by the Aztecs and Incas. The plant is cultivated largely in tropical regions, and where it grows, the leaves are eaten as a vegetable (they are similar in taste to spinach). The pale seed is highly nutritious, with more protein and oil content than many other grains, and tastes like nutty popcorn, with a peppery edge. When cooked, it becomes spongy and sticky. Amaranth is sold as a grain and a flour, and both are used frequently alongside other flours in bakes and snacks. Toasting the grains briefly before cooking helps them remain distinct.

NUTRITIONAL BENEFITS
A good source of protein, fibre, iron and calcium.

SERVING SUGGESTIONS
Cook the seeds in three times their volume of salted water or vegan milk for 20–25 minutes to make amaranth porridge; pop the grains in a hot, dry pan and add them to bread dough, granola or muesli, scatter over salads, or season and eat as a snack; add amaranth flour to flatbread dough; use instead of (or with) red lentils to make dhal.

TAPIOCA

This pale, starchy product is made from the dried root of the tropical American shrub, cassava, which is now mainly grown in Asia and Africa. It is available in flake form, granulated (ground flakes) and as pearled tapioca, and has a neutral flavour. Its maligned reputation as a bland English milk pudding has done it no favours, but – cooked well – its translucent, jelly-like quality can be an asset. In Brazilian cooking, tapioca is boiled or baked to make savoury and sweet dishes.

NUTRITIONAL BENEFITS
Negligible source of nutrients.

SERVING SUGGESTIONS
Cook pearl tapioca with coconut milk, sweeten and add vanilla, then serve as a pudding, with fruit; add tapioca starch to soups or sauces to thicken them; add tapioca starch to pancake batters; make puffed tapioca crackers.

tip

Powdered tapioca (also known as tapioca starch) is a useful binding and thickening agent in vegan diets, and the pearled product makes a soothing pudding.

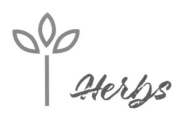

Herbs

The aromatic leaves of fresh or dried plants have been cherished for medicinal, ceremonial and culinary purposes for thousands of years. In the kitchen, they offer aroma, flavour and vibrancy and are used to perk up dishes and invigorate the palate. They are most often classified as belonging to either the carrot or the mint family – those in the carrot family have delicate leaves, and herbs of the mint family are more robust. They are best when eaten fresh, as their aromatic properties diminish quickly after picking. (The nutritional benefits correspond to fresh herbs, not dried.)

PARSLEY

One of the most ubiquitous and most versatile fresh culinary herbs in America and Europe, parsley brightens countless savoury dishes. Native to Mediterranean parts of southern Europe and western Asia, it was held in high esteem by the ancient Greeks for its reviving properties and is now cultivated across most temperate regions. The soft, vivid green herb has a strong, grassy aroma and tangy, mildly bittersweet flavour and is particularly nutritious, containing high quantities of vitamin C. Flat-leaf parsley is generally considered to have a superior and gutsier taste than curly-leaf, and is used in abundant quantities in Middle Eastern salads, notably tabbouleh. In France it is the key ingredient in French *fines herbes* (a blend of chervil, tarragon and chives) and *persillade*, and the stalks frequently appear in a bouquet garni. Chopping

parsley enhances its fresh, green flavours – the delicate leaves are best cooked only briefly, if at all. Chop parsley stalks finely for a salad or dressing, or add them to a vegetable soup or stock. Dried parsley has little flavour.

NUTRITIONAL BENEFITS
A good source of vitamins A and C, B vitamins, calcium and iron.

SERVING SUGGESTIONS
Stir chopped parsley and capers into a warm lentil or bean salad; chop and mix into crushed, steamed celeriac; add chopped parsley to a mushroom paté; make a gremolata with lemon zest, chopped parsley and garlic and sprinkle over roasted carrots; add stalks to a pot for cooking dried beans; make parsley oil, blitzing chopped leaves with garlic and olive oil; toss generous handfuls of chopped parsley with a little cooked bulgur wheat, tomatoes, spring onions, lemon juice, oil, garlic and mint to make *tabbouleh* salad.

BASIL

Thought to be native to tropical Asia, this highly aromatic and delicate herb is now cultivated in warm climates worldwide and has been used in Italian and Thai cuisines for centuries. Different varieties of the plant have distinct flavours, and are rarely interchangeable: sweet basil is the most common variety in Mediterranean cooking, and suits both sweet and savoury dishes. The soft green (sometimes purple) leaves have a sweet and grassy flavour with a sharp and anise edge, work well in sauces, dressings and salads and are a key ingredient in Italian pesto and its many southern European variants. The leaves are usually added at the end of cooking or served fresh, as prolonged heat causes their flavour to rapidly diminish. Handle the leaves with care, as they bruise easily – tearing them rather than chopping them causes less bruising. Dried basil is a poor reflection of the fresh herb.

THAI SWEET BASIL: Also known as Asian basil, Thai sweet basil has purple stems and a more pungent anise flavour than sweet basil. Large quantities of leaves are used in curries, salads and stir-fries (the leaves tolerate heat better than sweet basil).

HOLY BASIL: A variety of sweet basil with narrower, serrated leaves. It has a lemony scent and peppery clove-like flavour and is popular in Southeast Asian cuisines, particularly curries.

NUTRITIONAL BENEFITS
A good source of vitamins A, K and C and minerals.

SERVING SUGGESTIONS
Scatter fresh basil leaves over a tomato salad or tomato pasta dish; make a *salsa verde* with parsley, mint, basil, garlic, spring onions and capers, chopped together before stirring in olive oil – drizzle over new potatoes or roasted vegetables; use Thai basil in a coconut, spinach and aubergine curry; make a lime and sugar syrup, infuse with basil and drizzle over strawberries or freeze to make a granita.

CHIVES

This delicate member of the onion family is descended from a plant that grows wild in central Europe and Asia and has been cultivated in Europe since the sixteenth century for culinary use. The bright green hollow leaves have a subtle oniony bite, succulent texture and mild sweetness and are primarily used raw as a garnish for savoury dishes in the cuisines of Central and northern Europe. Chives also feature as one of the classic four *fines herbes* (along with

parsley, chervil and tarragon) used as a seasoning in French cooking. They lose most of their flavour when cooked and their flavour dissipates soon after cutting, so they should be used while at their freshest. Their pale lilac flowers share the leaves' delicate flavour (see box on page 143).

CHINESE CHIVES: These have a stronger garlic flavour than European chives and are sometimes called garlic chives (or 'kuchai'). The flat leaves are larger than regular chives, and the flowers are white. They are cooked in China, Japan and east Asia in the style of a vegetable rather than a herb.

NUTRITIONAL BENEFITS
A good source of vitamins A and C, B vitamins and minerals.

SERVING SUGGESTIONS
Snip chives and use as a garnish for a lettuce and pea soup; stir chopped chives into a cool broad bean dip or an avocado and bulgur wheat or bean salad; garnish asparagus risotto with snipped chives; scatter them over crushed new potatoes; snip Chinese chives and add to a tofu scramble or stir-fry; sprinkle snipped chives over spiced Jamaican rice and peas.

CORIANDER

Native to southern Europe and the Mediterranean region, this distinctive herb is indispensable in Latin, Indian and most Asian cuisines. Known as cilantro in North America, coriander has broad, flat leaves similar to flat-leaf parsley (the two herbs are related) and is considered an acquired taste: some describe it as 'soapy' and take a keen dislike to it, others adore it. It certainly has a complex flavour, incorporating earthiness and woody, pine-like notes with a cool, floral edge. Every part of the plant is edible, including the root, which is ground with the tender, aromatic stems in Thai and Indian cooking and added to spice pastes for stews, soups and curries. Asian grocers are the best place to look for the whole plant, and it's worth heading to one for the leaves too, as you get more for your money. The stems carry a lot of flavour and can be used in spice pastes and stocks. The delicate leaves are mainly used fresh or added at the end of cooking. (For the spice, see page 146.)

NUTRITIONAL BENEFITS
A good source of B vitamins and folic acid.

SERVING SUGGESTIONS
Use it as a salad leaf, in larger quantities than typical soft-leaf herbs, along with cooked grains and a punchy dressing; blitz with toasted peanuts, almonds, walnuts or hazelnuts to make a pesto; use coriander root and stems in Asian curry paste or South Indian dhal; stir chopped coriander into a dhal or tofu noodle soup; make a fresh Indian coconut and coriander chutney; make a North African chermoula paste with coriander, garlic, preserved lemon, olive oil, cumin and cayenne and use to baste grilled vegetables or drizzle over a black bean soup; make a coriander, lime and tomato salsa; team with avocado in a guacamole; stir chopped coriander through a Mexican bean stew just before serving.

MINT

Native to southern Europe and the Mediterranean, mint was a garden herb of great repute in ancient Greece and Rome. Today, its refreshing menthol flavour is recognized the world over, and of the hundreds of varieties of edible mint, spearmint and peppermint are the most widely used. Spearmint, the milder and sweeter of the two, with its green pointed leaves, is the key culinary herb, and the dark leaves of fiery peppermint are largely cultivated for making oil. In Chinese, Indian, Japanese, Malaysian and Thai cuisines, spearmint and closely related varieties are made into chutneys, sauces and drinks, and combined with other herbs: in North Africa and the Middle East, spearmint or dried peppermint are brewed with hot water to make tea. Mint's fresh, cooling effect and citrusy notes suit both savoury and sweet dishes. They are best added at the end of cooking, or eaten raw. Use dried mint during cooking but add fresh at the end.

NUTRITIONAL BENEFITS
A source of iron and minerals, and vitamins C and A.

SERVING SUGGESTIONS
Sprinkle chopped leaves over a melon, mango or pineapple salad; mix into vegan yoghurt with grated cucumber to make a raita for serving with curry or grilled aubergine; add to Vietnamese spring rolls, along with coriander; stir into a broad bean or pea dip; make mint sorbet; make a coconut and mint chutney with onion, chillies and freshly grated coconut; stir chopped parsley, mint and coriander through a quinoa pilaf; tear leaves and sprinkle over a Vietnamese noodle soup; add to the cooking water for new potatoes; scatter chopped leaves over a roasted beetroot borani.

DILL

Native to southern Europe and western Asia, dill – a member of the parsley family – grows wild in Spain, Portugal and Italy and is cultivated in numerous mild climates in the northern hemisphere. The plant's name is thought to stem from the Old Norse word *dilla*, meaning 'to lull', and it has been appreciated for the curative and aromatic properties of its foliage and seeds for millennia. Since the Middle Ages, dill's fragrant, feathery green fronds have become a common culinary herb in the cuisines of Scandinavia, Russia and the Ukraine, where their freshness and clean anise taste gently invigorates pickles, fish and other savoury dishes. It appears frequently in Greece, too, and in Turkey, Iran and northern Vietnam. Dill loses its aroma during cooking, so add it at the end, or use it raw. Dill seeds have a stronger flavour than the herb (see page 149). The sweetness of the fresh herb is lost when it's dried – use fresh where possible.

NUTRITIONAL BENEFITS
A good source of vitamins A and C and minerals.

SERVING SUGGESTIONS
Scatter over a warm new potato salad or beetroot soup; sprinkle over pickled cucumber or add it to a dressing to drizzle over a cucumber salad; stir through a Thai-spiced vegetable broth; make a creamy dressing with avocado, lemon and dill; combine grilled mushroom and quinoa,

buckwheat or bulgur wheat with a combination of dill and other chopped fresh herbs; stir fresh dill through a broad bean pilaf.

TARRAGON

Native to southeast Europe and Central Asia, tarragon became popular as a salad herb only in the sixteenth century, primarily in France and Central Europe (it's little used elsewhere). It is known as a key ingredient in béarnaise sauce, one of the key herbs in the delicate *fines herbes* mixture – a cornerstone of classic French cooking – and used to infuse vinegar. The liquorice scent of the slender green leaves shares similarities with fennel, and the flavour combines sharp anise with a mild sweetness. Avoid Russian tarragon (also known as false tarragon), which has a coarser texture and taste than the fragile French variety, by checking the packet. As with most other soft herbs, it should only be added near the end of cooking, to retain its fresh flavour, or used raw, though use it judiciously as it has an assertiveness and pungency that can overwhelm other flavours. Dried tarragon doesn't share the rich aromatic character of the fresh herb.

NUTRITIONAL BENEFITS
A good source of iron and minerals.

SERVING SUGGESTIONS
Stir a little chopped tarragon into a courgette risotto; add chopped tarragon to a dressing for roasting beetroots or whole artichokes; scatter over slow-roasted tomatoes or a fresh tomato salad; sprinkle chopped leaves over a warm green bean salad with toasted nuts and pickled shallots; infuse sugar syrup with tarragon then drizzle over a tropical fruit salad, or scatter chopped leaves over grilled peaches or nectarines.

OREGANO

Native to Europe and Central Asia, oregano is a wild variety of marjoram, with similar aromatic properties and culinary uses. The small, aromatic, kite-shaped leaves have been appreciated and cultivated for their heady aroma and peppery, savoury flavour since ancient times in the Mediterranean and Middle East and more recently in Latin America. Varieties grown in Greece and Sicily are considered particularly aromatic and pungent. The leaves have a slightly bitter taste and a warm spiciness that intensifies when the herb is dried, so use the dried herb in small quantities. The fresh herb and dried herb both suit robust savoury dishes, particularly ones in which vegetables are grilled and roasted. Add fresh oregano to dishes towards the end of cooking if you want to retain its floral character.

NUTRITIONAL BENEFITS
A good source of vitamin K and minerals.

SERVING SUGGESTIONS
Add a pinch of dried oregano to a tomato and aubergine bake; scatter over pizza or vegan Bolognese; make a Sicilian *salmoriglio* dressing with oregano, lemon and parsley; add fresh oregano to ribollita (Italian cabbage and bean soup); make a dressing with oregano, olive oil, garlic, and lemon juice and toss through cooked borlotti beans while they are still warm; stir dried oregano through an orzo and roast vegetable salad or Mexican bean chilli.

ROSEMARY

This hardy shrub, native to the Mediterranean, has long been admired and cultivated in kitchen gardens for the warm resinous scent of its leaves and flowers (see 143). It was initially appreciated for its medicinal and fragrant qualities rather than its culinary potential, before finding favour in European cuisines, particularly the food of Italy. The narrow, glossy leaves resemble pine needles and are strongly aromatic, with a bitter and complex taste that – like other woody herbs – works well with robust ingredients and suits both sweet and savoury dishes. Discard the stems and very finely chop the leaves before adding them to a dish, or add whole sprigs and remove the sprigs before serving, and use it in moderation as it is a pungent and assertive herb. It can withstand longer cooking than softer herbs.

NUTRITIONAL BENEFITS
A good source of vitamins A and C, B vitamins and minerals.

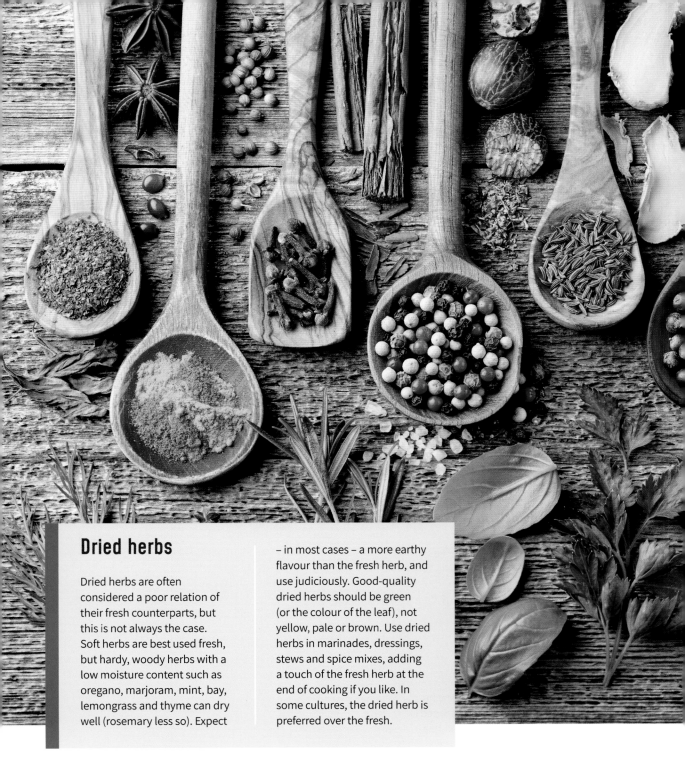

Dried herbs

Dried herbs are often considered a poor relation of their fresh counterparts, but this is not always the case. Soft herbs are best used fresh, but hardy, woody herbs with a low moisture content such as oregano, marjoram, mint, bay, lemongrass and thyme can dry well (rosemary less so). Expect – in most cases – a more earthy flavour than the fresh herb, and use judiciously. Good-quality dried herbs should be green (or the colour of the leaf), not yellow, pale or brown. Use dried herbs in marinades, dressings, stews and spice mixes, adding a touch of the fresh herb at the end of cooking if you like. In some cultures, the dried herb is preferred over the fresh.

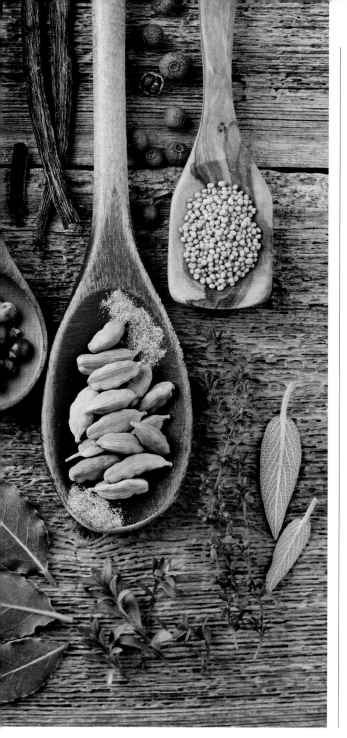

Make rosemary and blackberry, or rosemary and apricot jam; make rosemary salt and scatter over grilled or roasted vegetables; add a sprig to the pot when cooking beans such as cannellini, borlotti, haricot or kidney beans; add finely chopped rosemary to a crumb and toasted nut coating for aubergines, courgettes or halved tomatoes, before roasting; make a rosemary-infused sugar syrup to drizzle over lemon and almond cake; add sprigs to home-made lemonade; use the stripped stems as skewers for vegetable kebabs; toast almonds with rosemary.

THYME

Thyme flourishes in the wild on the arid hillsides of southern Europe and the Mediterranean and has been cherished for thousands of years for its aromatic qualities. Many dozens of cultivated varieties are used throughout the world, with 'common thyme' being the most widely known and versatile (with lemon thyme not far behind). Its small, soft, grey-green leaves are sharp, warm and spicy on the tongue and have a heady resinous scent. Where many hardy herbs can overwhelm other flavours, thyme is less pungent and works well in slow-cooked dishes. It is used in Spanish, French, South American and Mexican stews, marinades, herb and spice blends (such as Middle Eastern za'atar) and bouquet garni: it sits well with sweet flavours too. Strip the leaves from the stems before using, or add whole sprigs to a dish and remove before serving. Thyme dries well. (See also, edible flowers 143.)

NUTRITIONAL BENEFITS
A good source of vitamins C and A and minerals.

SERVING SUGGESTIONS
Add thyme leaves to an onion and garlic base for a slow-cooked tomato sauce; add thyme to an olive oil, lemon and garlic marinade for barbecued vegetables (try cauliflower, courgettes, red peppers or aubergines); add thyme leaves to the caramel for a pear or apple tart tatin made with vegan puff pastry; add sprigs of thyme to a lentil or bean stew; sprinkle thyme leaves into a ratatouille; fry mushrooms with thyme sprigs, then discard the sprigs; add a few thyme leaves to orange marmalade.

SAGE

A little goes a long way with this potent herb. Native to the north Mediterranean, sage is cultivated in temperate climates around the world and thrives in particularly dry, hot regions. It was admired for its medicinal virtues in ancient and medieval times, coming into use as a culinary herb and popular kitchen garden plant around the sixteenth century. Hundreds of varieties of sage, ranging from musky purple sage to delicate clary sage and pineapple sage, are used in cooking. 'Common sage', with its green to silver-grey leaves, is the type you're most likely to find in the supermarket. It is a key ingredient in northern Italian savoury cooking, where it is often paired in dishes with meat. German and British savoury dishes have long featured this punchy herb, too. Its velvety leaves have a spicy, citrus-and-pine quality and a bitter aftertaste. Its astringency means it lends itself well to oily, rich dishes, and it's one of the few herbs that dries well. Use sparingly. For the edible flowers, see 143.

NUTRITIONAL BENEFITS
A good source of vitamins A and K, and minerals.

SERVING SUGGESTIONS
Fry chopped shallots with shredded Brussels sprouts and sage leaves in oil then serve with pasta; fry sage leaves in oil and drizzle the sage-scented oil over roasted pumpkin or butternut squash, along with toasted pine nuts; add sage to chestnut soup; make an apple and sage jelly for serving with porridge; make an Italian haricot or borlotti bean stew, with sage, bay leaves and garlic.

BAY

Native to the eastern Mediterranean region, this hardy herb was considered sacred in ancient Greece, and appreciated for its culinary and medicinal qualities. Its heady perfume has held a pivotal role in cooking throughout Europe and the Mediterranean right up to the present day. The gentle resinous character of the aromatic, shiny, dark green leaves suits both savoury and sweet dishes and they are a key ingredient in many French and Mediterranean broths, soups and stews. Use them

to infuse dishes – the leathery leaves aren't pleasant to eat raw. Added whole or torn at the start of cooking, they gradually disperse their fragrance. They are essential to a bouquet garni, and are often added to pickles. Use the leaves sparingly.

NUTRITIONAL BENEFITS
A good source of vitamin A, B vitamins, calcium, iron and minerals.

SERVING SUGGESTIONS
Add leaves to braised courgettes; add to leek and potato soup; thread whole leaves onto vegetable skewers for barbecuing or grilling; add a couple of leaves to rhubarb before baking; add a whole leaf to an apple compote; throw a couple of leaves into poaching liquor for quinces, plums, pears or peaches; add to a berry jam; infuse the cooking water for polenta with a few bay leaves; add to a stock for an asparagus risotto; cook soaked cannellini beans in water with bay leaves; add to coconut rice pudding or a caramel sauce.

CURRY LEAVES

Curry leaves grow on a small tropical tree native to the foothills of the Himalayas and are now cultivated in southern India, the Middle East, Asia and northern Australia. The plant is a member of the citrus family and the dark green leaves are highly fragrant, with a mild lemony scent. When crushed or cut, the scent becomes floral, warm and complex. Curry leaves are used in abundance in the cuisines of coastal and southern India, Malaysia and Sri Lanka, their subtle character imparting a unique aromatic note to curries and dhals, pickles, chutneys and savoury relishes. They are crushed into spice pastes and often fried briefly in oil with spices until they crackle, to make a *tarka/tadka* (tempering), then stirred into vegetarian curries and dhals. Seek out fresh blemish-free leaves, sold on the stem, as dried leaves are significantly less aromatic (you can store any unused fresh leaves in the freezer). Their subtle flavour means they can be used liberally.

NUTRITIONAL BENEFITS

A good source of calcium, iron, minerals, B vitamins and vitamins A, C and E.

SERVING SUGGESTIONS

Fry fresh leaves in oil with mustard seeds before stirring into a dhal or chaat masala; add to the spice base for a butternut squash and aubergine curry, along with mustard seeds, cumin and ginger, before adding the vegetables and coconut milk; add chopped leaves to flatbread dough or scatter fried leaves over cooked flatbread; add to a pan of rice during cooking.

MAKRUT LIME LEAVES

Native to Southeast Asia, the tree that produces these aromatic leaves, also known as Thai lime leaves, belongs to a species of citrus. Makrut lime leaf gives savoury Thai, Cambodian and Indonesian dishes, particularly soups, broths and stews, a distinctive astringent, sour-citrusy flavour and aroma. They are hard to find fresh outside Southeast Asia, but can be found frozen in Asian or Chinese food shops (the dried leaves are an acceptable substitute). Fresh leaves are usually bruised, torn or shredded to help release their aromatic properties, but dried leaves do not require this. As with bay leaves, they are primarily used to infuse liquids and are not eaten raw: they also work in sweet dishes. The fragrant skin from the tree's dimpled green fruit is often added to dishes along with the leaves.

NUTRITIONAL BENEFITS

A good source of vitamin C, B vitamins and minerals.

SERVING SUGGESTIONS

Add the dried leaves to a Thai vegetable broth, along with lemongrass and ginger or galangal; infuse a sugar syrup with the leaves then use to make a lime sorbet; blitz (after removing the central ribs from the leaves) with Thai basil, soy sauce, sugar, garlic and spring onions to make a spice paste base for a stir-fry; pound fresh leaves with sugar and sprinkle over a tropical fruit salad.

LEMONGRASS

Lemongrass is cultivated throughout warm, tropical climates and is thought to be native to South India, Sri Lanka and Malaysia, where it has been used for both medicinal and culinary purposes for thousands of years, with Southeast Asian regions adopting it most enthusiastically as a spice. The narrow, tapering leaves grow from the bulbous plant base and have a distinct and delicate floral-citrus scent that enlivens curries, stir-fries, pickles, salads and soups, particularly in Thailand, Vietnam and Malaysia. The tender parts of the stalk are crushed or pounded in curry pastes and spice blends, and it adds a refreshing, peppery tang to rich, coconut-based curries and soups such as tom yum. Dried, ground lemongrass (often called 'sereh' powder) possesses only a fraction of the spice's complex character. Asian grocers tend to stock bundles of fresher, plumper lemongrass stalks than you'll find in supermarkets. The tender inner part of the stem can be eaten raw (finely diced or pounded). Lemongrass freezes well.

NUTRITIONAL BENEFITS

A good source of minerals.

SERVING SUGGESTIONS

Use the tender inner stalk in curry pastes, marinades and spice rubs; add finely chopped lemongrass to a dressing for a Thai noodle salad made with carrot, chilli, cucumber, toasted peanuts and plenty of coriander; add chopped lemongrass and ginger or galangal to sautéed shallots and garlic to lift a sweet potato soup or stir-fry; add to sugar syrup for poaching pears, rhubarb or peaches; don't throw away the woody tops of stalks – add them to the pan when cooking rice, stock or soup; use a gently bruised stalk to make tea, adding other aromatics such as lemon peel, ginger and a cinnamon stick.

tip

Bashing the fibrous stalk of lemongrass helps release its aromatics.

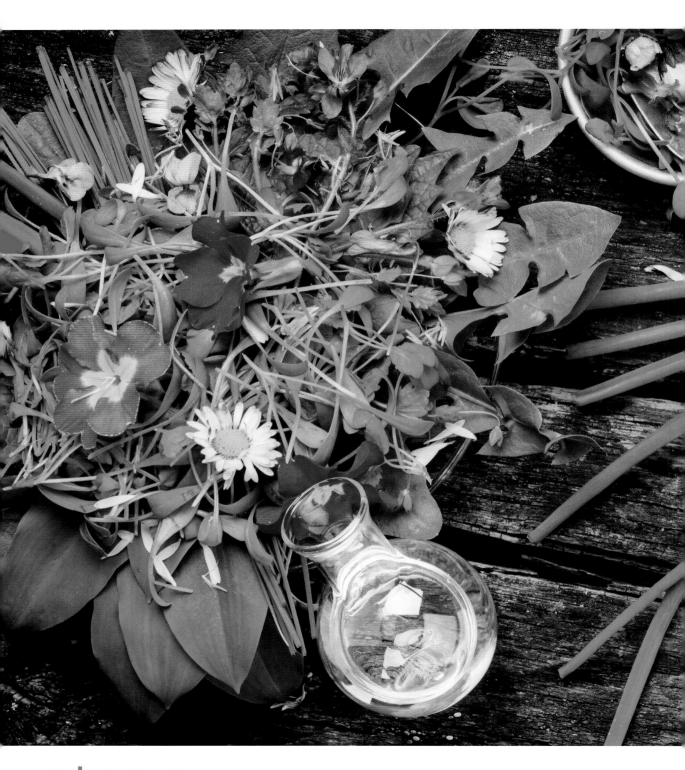

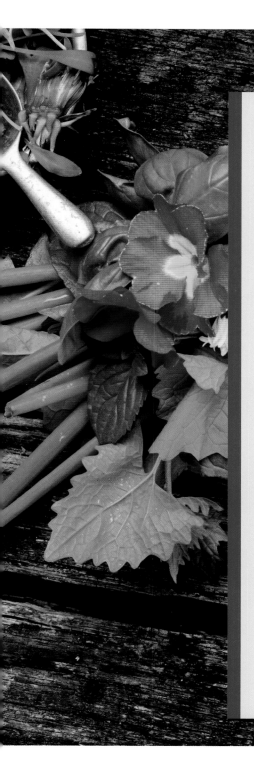

Edible flowers

Flowers from fresh herbs and kitchen gardens have long been used to perfume and decorate sweet and savoury dishes. Some are even substantial enough to be cooked whole (see courgette flowers on page 55).

The flowers from herb plants share a similar flavour profile to the herb, but have a more delicate, subtle taste.

Try adding one of these blossoms, or a combination, to salads, use as a garnish for a green vegetable stir-fry, add to jams or jellies, fry whole in batter, crystallize, make flavoured sugars for baking or infuse sugar syrups for making confectionary and granitas, or add to teas and infusions.

Note: be sure to use only unsprayed flowers that you have grown yourself, or flowers that are sold for culinary use.

Apple blossom

Basil flowers

Borage flowers

Calendula (marigold) flowers

Chive flowers (and garlic chive flowers)

Chrysanthemums

Corn flowers

Courgette flowers

Dahlias

Daisies

Dandelions

Dianthus

Dill flowers

Elderflower

Forget-me-nots

Hibiscus

Jasmine

Lavender

Nasturtium (flowers and leaves)

Pansies

Pea flowers

Primroses

Primulas

Roses

Rosemary flowers

Sage flowers

Snapdragons

Sweet woodruff

Thyme flowers

Oxalis

Violas

Violets

Wild garlic flowers

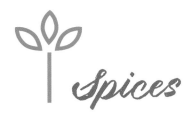

Spices

Spices have been used to enliven and enrich food with their evocative and intense flavours, and have acquired symbolic and therapeutic significance over thousands of years. The fragrant seeds, fruits, stems, flowers and barks mainly hail from tropical climates and are typically sold in their dry form. Many whole spices benefit from being toasted lightly before being crushed, to help release their aromatic oils.

TURMERIC

Turmeric, a musky, earthy spice in the ginger family, is thought to be native to India. The rhizome (a bulb-like underground stem) has been renowned since ancient times for its health-giving benefits and has long been used in Indian, Irani and North African cuisines. In Europe, it found popularity in all-purpose 'curry powder'. Turmeric is sold fresh, or dried and ground to a powder, and appreciated for its inviting yellow hue as well as for its pungent flavour. Use it sparingly to avoid its bitterness overwhelming other flavours. Adding black pepper to dishes containing turmeric increases the bioavailability of turmeric's curcumin. Ground turmeric loses its flavour rapidly: buy only in small quantities. Raw turmeric should be plump, not wrinkled, and can be frozen.

NUTRITIONAL BENEFITS
Fresh turmeric is a good source of vitamin C and minerals (manganese, iron and potassium)

SERVING SUGGESTIONS
Combine dried or freshly grated turmeric with mustard seeds and asafoetida in vegetable piccalilli-style pickles; grate fresh turmeric or add a pinch of ground turmeric to a vegetable and chickpea stew or North African pilaf with pistachios, cinnamon and green cardamom; add a pinch of turmeric to a savoury pastry dough; add crushed fresh turmeric to a chilli, garlic, lemongrass and galangal spice paste.

Galangal

The knobbly roots of this fibrous, peppery rhizome resemble ginger, but it is sweeter and milder. Native to Indonesia, galangal comes from a tropical plant in the ginger family and is used in Malaysia, Thailand and Indonesia to brighten hot-and-sour dishes, soups, laksas, sambals and curry pastes with its fragrant, citrusy warmth. Dried, ground galangal sometimes features in Middle Eastern and North African spice blends such as ras-el-hanout. Soak dried galangal slices in hot water before using, or use fresh sliced or grated galangal to flavour Asian soups and stews: add to a lime dressing for a papaya salad: swap ginger for galangal in a fruit or vegetable smoothie: or combine lemongrass and galangal in a Thai curry.

GINGER

This warming spice comes from a bamboo-like tropical plant native to tropical Asia and was one of the first oriental spices to reach Europe. For thousands of years it held a high status as a medicinal and culinary spice: dried ginger once had a place on European tables as a condiment and in the Middle Ages was widely used in savoury and sweet cooking, but it's now more commonly used as a dry baking spice. Dried ginger also appears in spice blends including *quatre epices*, ras-el-hanout and Chinese five-spice. In Asia fresh ginger is more commonly used. Fresh ginger has a citrusy tang and fresh heat, and dried ginger is woodier and more pungent. Use a teaspoon to scrape away the skin from fresh ginger, if it needs peeling. Fresh ginger can be frozen.

NUTRITIONAL BENEFITS
Vitamin C and minerals such as iron and potassium.

SERVING SUGGESTIONS
Add to stir-fries with garlic and shredded green cabbage; grate it into the oniony base for a rich, root-vegetable soup; add a generous grating of ginger to vegetable curries and dhals, or Asian-style slaws; add slices of fresh ginger to rhubarb or pears for poaching; add ground ginger to biscuit doughs; use fresh ginger in fruit or vegetable chutneys.

CHILLIES

Native to Mexico, Central and South America, this fruity, hot spice has been cultivated in these regions since around 7,000 BC, and only became known further afield when Columbus brought it to Europe in the late fifteenth century. From there, the Portuguese took chillies to India, Asia and Africa, where they quickly replaced black pepper as the most popular hot spice. They were embraced enthusiastically in Italian, Hungarian, Spanish and Portuguese kitchens, too. Chillies come in all shapes, sizes and colours and are appreciated for their flavour as much as for their heat, which can vary from mild and fruity to pungent and fiery hot. Once harvested, chillies are sold fresh (ripe or unripe), pickled or dried. In Mexican cooking, chillies of myriad varieties are grown (and often sun-dried) for distinct uses in pickles, relishes, sauces, stews and salsas. In Latin America, Asia, Africa and the Caribbean, chillies appear in countless spice blends and pastes, from Ethiopian *berbere* and North African harissa to Indian masalas and Indonesian *sambal olek*.

Typically, the smaller a chilli is, the hotter it is: some large, mild chillies can be cooked as a vegetable the tiniest should be used with caution. The white membrane inside chillies is the hottest part as it contains the highest levels of capsaicin, the source of spiciness. Wear gloves when handling fresh chillies. Whole dried chillies should be pliable, not brittle. Wipe them clean, remove the stems and seeds, dry-toast, then soak before using.

PAPRIKA: this sweet and fruity rust-red chilli powder is made from different varieties of chilli pepper, depending on where it is produced. Sometimes it is ground with seeds intact, to make a spicy product, but for most paprikas they are removed to make a mild (sweet) spice. Hungarian goulash isn't authentic unless it is made with paprika, and the powder is key to Spanish paella. In Spain, paprika is called *pimentón* and is available as *dulce* (sweet), *agridulce* (bittersweet) and *picante* (hot). Sweet paprika is often added at the start of cooking and hot used at the end. Some paprika is made with smoked chillies – smoked paprika from the La Vera valley region in Spain is highly prized. Turkish *pul biber*, semi-dried and roughly ground paprika chilli, is a popular spice in the Middle East, and the chilli often appears in fiery baharat spice mix. Paprika fried in oil will burn easily: instead, add it to cooking liquid or ingredients that have already been sautéed.

NUTRITIONAL BENEFITS
Chillies are a richer source of vitamin C than citrus fruits, and are rich in vitamin A, B vitamins and minerals.

SERVING SUGGESTIONS
Add fresh chilli to a fresh coconut relish to serve with grilled vegetables; dust chilli powder over a tropical fruit salad; sprinkle smoked chilli flakes over cool gazpacho or a cucumber and vegan yoghurt dip; make a peperonata with sweet peppers and hot chillies; add soaked, finely chopped dried chillies or fresh chillies to vegan cornbread or naan bread; add smoked dried chilli to Boston baked beans or refried beans; sprinkle chilli flakes over a tofu stir-fry; add smoked paprika to the tomato sauce for Spanish *patatas bravas* or corn chowder; sprinkle sweet paprika into a pan of sautéed onions for a paella or add to couscous before soaking it in water.

BLACK PEPPERCORNS

Perhaps the world's most ubiquitous spice, this classic seasoning, and salt's regular table companion, comes from a tropical climbing vine native to India's Malabar coast. Known as the 'king of spices' this pungent, warm and woody spice has been a precious commodity since antiquity. Today, it is a familiar sight in the western kitchen, ground mainly over savoury foods as a flavour enhancer (though it also works well with sweet foods). It is intrinsic to many spice mixes, including garam masala and Middle Eastern baharat spice blends. Buy higher-quality pepper and you will notice complex, floral and fruity notes in addition to the heat. As a rule, the bigger the peppercorns, the better they taste. Buy peppercorns whole and grind as needed.

White peppercorns are an essential ingredient in classic French sauces and have a more delicate taste than black peppercorns.

Green peppercorns, available fresh, bottled in brine or freeze-dried, are popular in Thai cuisine, particularly curries, and French patés and terrines, and their heat is more herbaceous than black peppercorns'. Rinse brined peppercorns before using.

NUTRITIONAL BENEFITS
A good source of minerals, B vitamins and vitamin K.

SERVING SUGGESTIONS
Add whole black or green peppercorns to a brine for preserving roasted red peppers or cucumber: add a few grinds to an onion marmalade; sprinkle freshly ground pepper over peaches, nectarines, melon or watermelon; macerate fresh strawberries with sugar and a little black pepper, then use to make a sorbet; add a generous grind of black pepper to savoury pastry dough; lightly toast the peppercorns, then grind and add to a South Indian vegetable curry.

CORIANDER SEEDS

Coriander 'seeds' are a fruit from a plant in the parsley family native to the Mediterranean and southern Europe. The whole plant is edible and the leaves are used as a herb (see page 135). Coriander seeds were used by the ancient Greeks and Romans as a medicine, preservative and culinary spice, and have been a signature spice in North Indian cuisines for thousands of years. The seeds have a floral and bittersweet taste and are often used in combination with other spices: it is a key component of all-purpose curry powders, Georgian *khmeli suneli*, Arab baharat, North African harissa, Ethiopian *berbere*, Egyptian *taklia* and Moroccan ras-el-hanout. The brittle seeds are easy to crush. Dry-toast them lightly before using to intensify their sweet citrusy notes.

NUTRITIONAL BENEFITS
A good source of vitamin C and minerals.

SERVING SUGGESTIONS
Toss a few crushed seeds through a cabbage and apple slaw or sprinkle over sautéed greens; add crushed coriander seeds to a Mediterranean vegetable stew of aubergines, courgettes, tomatoes, peppers and onions;

add a few crushed coriander seeds to a sweet crumble mixture before scattering over apples; combine with other warm spices in the base for a curried lentil soup; add to rye bread dough; add to a tomato chutney or relish.

CUMIN SEEDS

These delicate, parchment-coloured seeds (fruit) come from a plant in the parsley family thought to be native to Egypt and the eastern Mediterranean. Cumin seeds found in Egypt's pyramids allude to their culinary and medicinal value, and it's known that it was used alongside salt as a condiment in ancient Rome. Today, the distinctive, highly aromatic and pungent flavour of cumin features in many spice blends, including all-purpose curry powders, Middle East baharat, Indian garam masala and *panch phoran*, Afghanistan's char masala and Moroccan ras-el-hanout. It is also features in many of Mexico's signature dishes. Ground cumin and coriander is a classic combination in the curries, pilafs and soups of north of India and Sri Lanka. Dry-toast whole seeds or roast them in oil to mellow the spice and enhance its lemony taste.

NUTRITIONAL BENEFITS
A good source of minerals, particularly iron.

SERVING SUGGESTIONS
Sprinkle ground cumin over cauliflower before roasting; dry-toast and crush the seeds and sprinkle them over a beetroot dip, hummus or baba ganoush; add a pinch of ground cumin to dhal and lentil stews; add a pinch of ground cumin to a falafel mixture, or base for a pilaf; fry tinned, drained black beans in oil with ground cumin then use to fill tacos or burritos; sprinkle a pinch of cumin over coconut yoghurt raita.

MUSTARD SEEDS

Mustard plants belong to the cabbage family and three main types are cultivated for different culinary purposes. Pale yellow seeds (called white mustard) are native to the Mediterranean and are cultivated in Canada mainly for use in pickling and American mustard, the spicier brown seeds are cultivated in India for cooking with and adding to spice

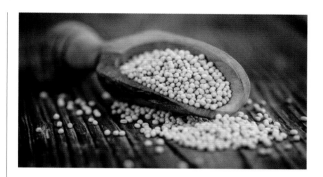

blends and pickles, and the black, a component of Bengali *panch phoran* spice mix, are less common and the most fiery. Mustard is an ancient spice, long admired for its curative qualities and pulverized to use as a condiment. It has no scent – the pungent heat is only released when the seeds are crushed and mixed with liquids such as oil, vinegar or water. Blended mustards such as Dijon mustard, and mustard powders, have been made in Europe and America for many centuries. Prolonged heat reduces prepared mustard's pungency so it is normally added at the end of cooking.

NUTRITIONAL BENEFITS
A good source of minerals and omega-3 fats.

SERVING SUGGESTIONS
Fry brown mustard seeds in ghee with other warm spices as a base for a cauliflower, okra or potato curry, or stir into dhal; add a spoon of wholegrain or Dijon mustard to a leek or Jerusalem artichoke bake; combine English mustard powder with black treacle and add to home-made baked beans; add mustard to a dressing for potato salad; add white mustard seeds to a pickled lemon relish, or the brine for a crisp vegetable pickle.

CARDAMOM

Green cardamom, a member of the ginger family, is native to the tropical forests of southern India and Sri Lanka. The firm, dry seed pods contain between twelve and twenty fragrant seeds. It is considered the 'Queen of Spices' (the 'King' being black pepper), and its intense citrusy-sweet and pungent aroma and taste has beguiled

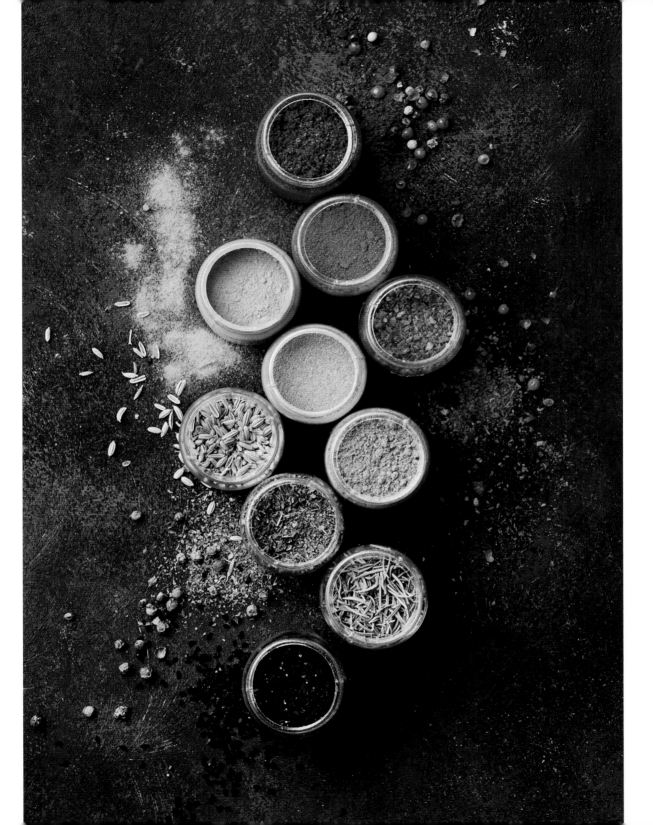

cooks and physicians for millennia. It is the third most expensive spice after saffron and vanilla, and an essential ingredient in a multitude of Indian sweet and savoury dishes and spice blends, and the Middle Eastern *gahwa* (spiced coffee). Scandinavians use it plentifully in breads and pastries, too. Use whole pods for a subtle flavour (removing them before serving) or crush the seeds in a pestle and mortar for a more potent hit. The black seeds inside the pods stale quickly, so grind as required.

Black cardamom: Native to the eastern Himalayas, black cardamom is a dried and cured leathery seed pod that contains resinous black-brown seeds. It is larger than green cardamom and has a distinct smoky flavour profile so one shouldn't be substituted for the other (it doesn't work with sweet foods). It is used in South Asian and Indian slow-cooked savoury dishes, in Sichuan braises, Vietnamese soups and Nepalese spice mixes and appreciated for its camphorous, earthy taste.

NUTRITIONAL BENEFITS
A good source of minerals (particularly iron).

SERVING SUGGESTIONS
Grind black cardamom seeds and sprinkle them over whole roasted cauliflower; fry crushed black cardamom seeds with other warming spices for a fragrant pilaf or dhal; sprinkle a little crushed green cardamom over a fruit jelly, or a sweet apple bake; toast green cardamom pods lightly in oil, then add rice for a pilaf; poach apricots with green cardamom; sprinkle a little crushed green cardamom over baked carrots or sweet potatoes.

NIGELLA SEEDS

These small, hard matt-black seeds are sometimes called black cumin, black onion seed (*kalonji*) and black sesame, though nigella isn't related to any of these spices. They come from seed pods that resemble a poppy head, and are native to southern Europe, Western Asia and the Middle East. They have a mild scent and a complex, peppery and herbaceous flavour that teams well with other spices, particularly coriander and allspice. The spice has been cultivated since ancient times, for therapeutic

use and in baking and pickling. It is one of the five spices in Bengali *panch phoran* spice mix, and is often added to the Middle Eastern dukkah spice mix. Dry-toasting emphasizes its subtle flavour and aroma.

NUTRITIONAL BENEFITS
A good source of minerals.

SERVING SUGGESTIONS
Dry-toast or fry lightly in oil with other spices and sprinkle over potato and cauliflower curry or dhal; add to vegetarian root-vegetable curries, baked aubergines, or grain salads; toss a pinch of nigella seeds with par-boiled potatoes or carrots before roasting; sprinkle nigella seeds over a butter bean dip or on flatbreads, naan breads, savoury biscuits and sweet cakes before or after baking; use the seeds as a pickling spice in chutneys or preserved lemon; add to stir-fried cabbage.

SUMAC

Sumac belongs to the cashew family and grows across the Mediterranean and Middle East and in some parts of Asia. The dried, rust-coloured berries are usually ground but can also be found whole, dried and intact on their stalks, in sumac's growing areas. Its use as a souring agent, and appreciation of its colour, dates back to ancient times, and it has long been essential to the Middle Eastern *za'atar* spice blend. More recently, the tart spice has become a common sight in western pantries. It has a subtle aroma and its gentle astringency helps brings out the flavour of savoury foods much like salt and lemon do. It should be slightly moist. It loses its potency and astringency if cooked.

NUTRITIONAL BENEFITS
A good source of minerals.

SERVING SUGGESTIONS
Sprinkle onto a toasted pitta, tomato, cucumber and lettuce salad (fattoush) or warm couscous; mix with oil and use to dress a red onion relish; sprinkle over grilled courgettes, roasted root vegetables, aubergines, chard or spinach; sprinkle over fried chickpeas or use in spiced falafels; dust over pitta breads or flatbread pizzas.

CARAWAY SEEDS

These five-ridged, crescent-shaped seeds are sometimes mistaken for cumin seeds. Native to Central Europe and Asia, they have held medicinal, symbolic and culinary significance in these regions since ancient times. Caraway seed's complex anise-like peppery taste and robust flavour can be found in many Central European savoury dishes and it's an essential ingredient in Algerian and Tunisian spice blends and some North African harissas. It has been used in sweet and savoury baking and pickling for centuries, too: caraway and cabbage is a classic flavour combination, and it is a traditional addition to rye bread in Scandinavia and Eastern Europe. The seeds are best used whole, or ground as needed. Gentle toasting heightens their flavour.

NUTRITIONAL BENEFITS
A good source of minerals.

SERVING SUGGESTIONS
Sauté thinly sliced Savoy cabbage with a generous pinch of freshly ground caraway; add a pinch of freshly ground caraway to a carrot or beetroot soup; sprinkle it over roast cauliflower; add it to gingerbread dough, along with other warm spices and ground ginger; sprinkle a little over baked vegan shortbread.

FENNEL SEEDS

The whole of this hardy plant is aromatic, and it has been consumed as a vegetable (see page 80) and spice for thousands of years. Its native growing areas are southern Europe and the Mediterranean. Fennel seeds (the plant's fruits) were prescribed in ancient times for almost every malady, and in India candied seeds are often chewed after a meal to aid digestion. Their aniseedy bite brings warmth and freshness to rich dishes from Italy to India: they are a component of spice blends too, including Bengal's *panch phoran*, Chinese five-spice and Sri Lankan curry powder. The mild liquorice taste complements both sweet and savoury foods.

NUTRITIONAL BENEFITS
A good source of minerals.

tip

Avoid buying ground fennel: the seeds are soft and easy to grind, and retain their aroma better if used whole, toasted or ground as needed.

SERVING SUGGESTIONS
Add toasted seeds to fruit jam or sprinkle over baked pears or apples; add to a fresh fennel and cabbage slaw; add freshly ground seeds to the Sardinian vegetable dish *caponata*, made with aubergines, courgettes, celery, capers, olives and tomatoes; crush with cumin and sprinkle over potatoes and onions before roasting; add a pinch of seeds to flatbread dough; sprinkle over sweet pastry before or after baking; grind and mix with ground ginger and turmeric for a vegetable curry.

DILL SEEDS

Dill is a hardy, annual plant in the parsley family, related to cumin, caraway and coriander. The plant's seeds (fruit) and feathery, fern-like leaves (see page 136) share a similar warming yet refreshing aromatic profile. Native to southern Europe and western Asia, it has been credited with alleviating digestive complaints and used as a seasoning in vinegars and pickles, and as a spice, for many thousands of years. Scandinavians and central and eastern Europeans are particularly fond of it. The seeds hold their own in strongly flavoured dishes, but their fresh sweetness helps lighten dishes and breads, too. Dill is often paired with caraway in sauerkraut. Add at the end of cooking to retain its pungency. The seeds have little aroma until crushed.

NUTRITIONAL BENEFITS
A good source of vitamin C and minerals.

SERVING SUGGESTIONS
Add seeds to sautéed green cabbage; add toasted seeds to a creamy vegan dressing for a slaw or potato salad;

sprinkle the seeds over roasted carrots or baked onions; add a pinch into a pan with chopped root vegetables and crushed coriander and cumin seeds; toss par-boiled parsnip 'chips' with dill and garlic-salt before baking; add dill to a spice mix for dhal; fry the seeds in oil and brush over baked flatbread; make dill-seed rye bread; add the seeds to cracker or oatcake dough.

STAR ANISE

As the fruit of the star anise tree, a small evergreen tree native to southwestern China and northeastern Vietnam, ripens, it forms a star-shaped pod. Each of the pod's points (carpels) contains a shiny seed, but it is the woody carpel that is the most fragrant. The warm, liquorice-sweet spice has been synonymous with Chinese cuisine for millennia and is an essential component of five-spice powder. In South India and Vietnam, it is added to rice dishes and pho noodle soup. Used whole, the pods offer their distinctive flavour and a decorative element to a dish. Once ground, the spice loses its impact. European anise seeds share a similar flavour profile but are from an unrelated plant.

NUTRITIONAL BENEFITS
A good source of minerals.

SERVING SUGGESTIONS
Add whole star anise to the pot when sautéing cabbage or fennel; sprinkle freshly ground star anise over butternut squash, sweet potato or swede before roasting; add star anise to fruit preserves or cooked fruit for a crumble; impart star anise's fragrance to rice by adding a pod to the pan at the start of cooking; marinate tofu in five-spice and soy sauce, then slice and add to stir-fries or rice.

CINNAMON AND CASSIA

Cinnamon and cassia both come from small, tropical evergreen trees: cinnamon is native to Sri Lanka and cassia to southern China. Cinnamon is harvested from young tree shoots and has a more delicate taste than cassia bark, which is harvested from mature trees, and is darker and coarser, with a more potent, spicier flavour.

Cinnamon tends to lend itself better to sweet dishes, and cassia to savoury, though in North America both are used interchangeably in sweet bakes. Cinnamon itself doesn't taste sweet, but it helps bring out sweetness in other ingredients. In Africa and the Middle East, and their native growing areas, cinnamon and cassia are mainly used in savoury cooking, added early in the cooking process to allow time for the bark's flavour to infuse a dish. Ground cinnamon, however, should be added towards the end of cooking to avoid it becoming bitter.

NUTRITIONAL BENEFITS
A good source of minerals.

SERVING SUGGESTIONS
Sprinkle a sugar and ground cinnamon mix over soft fruits such as peaches or figs before baking or grilling, or over a fresh fruit salad; add a cinnamon stick to poached fruit; add ground cinnamon to a dressing for tabbouleh, along with other warm spices; infuse a tomato sauce with a cinnamon stick and serve with Egyptian *koshari* (a mix of cooked lentils, macaroni and rice); add a cinnamon stick or piece of cassia bark to the base aromatic ingredients for a pilaf, dhal or curry; sprinkle ground cinnamon over a vegan rice pudding or overnight oats.

NUTMEG

Native to the remote Banda Islands of Indonesia, the nutmeg kernel comes from a large seed (fruit) of a tropical evergreen tree. The seed is covered with a lacy aril, which is sold separately as mace. The Europeans insatiable appetite for the cherished spice triggered a race to find its source in the sixteenth century. It may no longer be so ubiquitous, but it remains a signature spice in many traditional European bakes, puddings and savoury dishes. Nutmeg's powerful, bittersweet and woody flavour lends itself to both sweet and savoury dishes. It takes well to being paired with other spices, too, particularly cinnamon, star anise, black pepper and cloves. Grate it over a dish at the end of the cooking process, or use in bakes.

NUTRITIONAL BENEFITS

A good source of minerals.

SERVING SUGGESTIONS

Grate nutmeg over cooked spinach or a butternut squash or pea soup; grate it into the mixture for vegan apple cake or muffins; grate into vegan béchamel for vegetable lasagne; sprinkle grated nutmeg over mashed potato; combine with other warm spices and sprinkle over a warm rice pudding.

SAFFRON

It takes more than 5,000 flowers to make 1oz of this precious spice. Harvesting the thread-like red stigmas of the crocus plant is a painstaking process. Native to parts of the Mediterranean, saffron has been grown and highly prized since the Early Bronze Age, for its vivid colour, its purported medicinal value and unique warm and penetrating flavour. A little goes a long way, so buy the best you can afford, from a reliable source (to avoid 'fake' saffron) – Kashmiri saffron and saffron from La Mancha in Spain are both highly regarded. Avoid ground saffron, as it is often adulterated with other ingredients. From Spain to northern India, North Africa and the Middle East to Central Asia, it is used to give sweet and savoury foods, particularly rice dishes, a rich golden hue and exotic, delicate aroma. Steep saffron in warm water or other cooking liquid and add it towards the end of cooking, or dry threads in a low oven until brittle, then grind or crumble over finished dishes.

NUTRITIONAL BENEFITS

A good source of vitamin B_2, vitamin C and minerals.

SERVING SUGGESTIONS

Add a pinch of saffron to earthy vegetable soups and stews; rehydrate couscous in saffron-infused water and serve with preserved lemon in a salad; or add a couple of strands to poaching liquid for pears, peaches or apricots; make a Spanish vegetable paella with saffron-infused stock; sprinkle saffron-infused water over a butternut squash or broad bean pilaf; add saffron-infused water or vegan milk to sweet bread doughs.

CLOVES

Clove's journey in the world of spice echoes that of nutmeg and mace, which are also native to the Indonesian Molucca islands (the archipelago of islands was known as the 'Spice Islands'). The dried flower buds are highly scented and have been admired for their perfume for thousands of years. They share similar warming flavour notes with cinnamon and allspice and are key to many spice blends, including garam masala, Chinese five-spice, *quatre epices*, baharat and mixed spice. Clove appears in many European sweet dishes, including spiced bakes, and in festive Christmas dishes, with India and China using it for more savoury purposes. It can overpower other flavours, so use it sparingly. When grinding cloves, only use the round top.

NUTRITIONAL BENEFITS

A good source of minerals and vitamin K.

SERVING SUGGESTIONS

Add a pinch of ground cloves to braised red cabbage and apple; add one or two whole cloves to the water when cooking rice (remove them before serving); add a small pinch of ground cloves to a carrot and lentil soup; team clove with pears, quinces or figs in desserts; add cloves to brine for pickled vegetables.

JUNIPER

Juniper berries are tiny seed cones from an evergreen shrub in the cypress family. From ancient times the purple-black resinous berries have been appreciated more keenly for their curative properties and as an air purifier than as a culinary spice. Most of the yield from modern-day juniper berry cultivation is destined for gin distilleries: juniper's use in drinks-making dates back to thirteenth-century Netherlands, where the berries were used to flavour spirits, a practice enthusiastically adopted by the English a few centuries later. Its use in food is closely associated with savoury dishes of the Alps, France, Germany, Italy and Scandinavia, particularly sauerkraut, in which it is often teamed with caraway. Juniper has a sweet, warming taste with a refreshing hint of pine. The dried berries are easy to crush: bruising them lightly helps release their fragrant oils.

NUTRITIONAL BENEFITS
A good source of minerals.

SERVING SUGGESTIONS
Braise red cabbage and apple with a little crushed juniper; sprinkle crushed berries mixed with a little salt over beetroots, Brussels sprouts or carrots before roasting; sprinkle a small pinch over lemon or lime sorbet; add a pinch of crushed berries to vegan chocolate truffles or sweet energy ball mixtures.

ALLSPICE

As its name suggests, this New World berry is a versatile spice that lends itself to sweet and savoury dishes equally well. Native to the West Indies and Central and South America, the fruit of the allspice tree is also known as Jamaican pepper, or *pimiento* in Spain, as it was mistaken for pepper by Christopher Columbus when he discovered the spice in Jamaica. Allspice was in use long before Columbus's arrival, however, particularly by Mayans and Caribbeans, for its healing and preservative qualities and to flavour chocolate drinks. Once it reached Europe and North America, it took hold as a curing and pickling agent, and a mulling spice. It is a cornerstone spice in Jamaica, and essential to jerk seasoning. Its mellow, warming, peppery flavour appears in the Middle Eastern *berbere* spice blend, too, and European baking. Buy whole dried berries and grind as required.

NUTRITIONAL BENEFITS
A good source of minerals.

SERVING SUGGESTIONS
Use with black peppercorns and white mustard seeds in pickling liquid for beetroots, carrots or cauliflower; team with bay leaves in beetroot borsch; crush a berry and add it to poached plums; sprinkle a little ground allspice over slow-roasted tomatoes; sprinkle over grilled pineapple; make Jamaican 'rice and peas'; add ground allspice to the oniony base for a Middle Eastern pilaf or South Indian biryani; add a pinch of ground allspice to a rich ginger cake; add ground allspice to a tomato and borlotti bean bake.

FENUGREEK

Native to southeastern Europe and western Asia, the fenugreek plant was considered a cure-all in ancient times when both its hard, amber-coloured seeds and fragrant leaves were consumed. In the Middle East, western Asia, India and Sri Lanka, fenugreek is used as a herb, vegetable and a bittersweet spice. Commercial curry powder's musky scent comes from fenugreek seed, and it features also in Ethiopia's *berbere* spice blend, South Indian and Sri Lankan *sambar*, and *panch phoran*. Lightly toast the seeds to mellow them and enhance their savoury flavour before crushing, or soaking in water, then pound to a paste: use in stews and curries to help thicken them. The seeds can also be sprouted (see page 95).

Fenugreek leaves: In India and Pakistan, East Africa and the Middle East, astringent fresh fenugreek leaves are known as *methi* and are a staple vegetable, often paired with potatoes. Dried fenugreek leaves are popular in Punjabi and Persian cooking and baking.

NUTRITIONAL BENEFITS
The seeds are a good source of calcium and minerals (particularly iron), and the fresh leaves are a rich source of minerals and vitamin C.

SERVING SUGGESTIONS
Add ground fenugreek to fruit chutneys and relishes; add sprouted seeds to a salad; add dried fenugreek leaves to a potato and cauliflower curry; sauté fenugreek seeds with mustard seeds and onions before adding red lentils to make a dhal; make a creamy curry with paneer or tofu, blitzed cashews or coconut milk and warm spices, adding dried fenugreek leaves or soaked seeds.

Vegan cheeses,
YOGHURTS, CREAMS & BUTTERS

For anyone adopting a vegan diet, finding alternatives to dairy cheese, yoghurt, cream and butter that hit the mark and can hold their own in terms of taste and texture can be a challenge. Fortunately, an increasing number of plant-based dairy-free alternatives are appearing on shop shelves, thanks to enterprising producers who are transforming grains, nuts and legumes into vegan-friendly products that are luxurious, creamy and satisfying in their own right.

Many plant-based dairy alternatives are fortified with vitamins and minerals, but contain less calcium and protein than dairy milk, so (as with vegan milks) ensure you are eating foods rich in calcium, iodine and protein to avoid a deficiency. Check product labels for nutritional information and keep an eye on sugar content: nut-dairy alternatives tend to be highly sweetened.

VEGAN CHEESES

Mimicking the texture of a hard cheese, and its complex umami taste, are the toughest challenges for the dairy-free market. Manufacturers and artisan producers use various plant sources, including nuts, soya and coconut, to make block 'cheese' for grating and melting, and creamier, softer products for spreading, and their methods and the resulting products vary widely. Both cultured and non-cultured varieties are available: cultured cheeses are mostly hard vegan cheeses made to substitute Cheddar and other strong-flavoured cheeses. Most commercially produced vegan cheeses are uncultured products made with added flavourings, thickeners, oils and acidifying agents, fortified with vitamin B_{12} and calcium. Vegan cheese-making kits, and vegan cheesemongers can be found online if you want to avoid synthetic additives.

HARD:
The best hard cheese substitutes are made using vegan bacterial culturing and ageing methods that mimic the dairy cheese-making process and produce a 'cheese' that has a similar acidity, complexity and tang to dairy cheese. Many hard vegan cheese melt well, and smoked versions are also available. Vegan Parmesan cheese is made with nutritional yeast (see box opposite), nuts and salt, which is blended to form a fine crumb, ready for sprinkling. Some artisan vegan cheeses qualify as worthy additions to a cheeseboard.

SOFT:
Non-dairy soft cheeses are typically made with coconut oil, thickeners, flavourings and added vitamins, though some products are now available that are made with fermented nut milks and natural flavourings and contain fewer (or no) artificial additives or preservatives. They can be used as alternatives to ricotta, feta, cream cheese, halloumi and mozzarella.

To make your own mild-flavoured soft spread, see page 168.

NON-DAIRY SPREADS

Plenty of vegan-friendly butter alternatives are on offer in the chilled aisle, and there's coconut oil (see page 113) which acts a lot like butter: it is solid at room temperature and melts when hot, and is a good substitute for butter in cooking. Olive oil spreads are good for shallow-frying, soya spreads for spreading, and sunflower spreads and avocado butters for baking. Be mindful that although margarines are vegetable-oil based butter substitutes, they often contain lactose or whey, so check labels carefully. When baking with non-dairy spreads, swap butter for the same quantity of unsalted vegan spread or margarine (blocks of vegetable shortening works best for crispy pastry). Most non-dairy spreads are fortified with added vitamins and minerals.

CREAMS

Products that mimic the smooth texture and taste of cream are typically made from oats, grains, nuts or soya beans, with added thickeners and artificial flavourings. They generally work well as substitutes for dairy in puddings, and are available sweetened and unsweetened. 'Squirty' vegan cream is also available. Organic coconut cream makes a good additive-free substitution for dairy cream.

Try these methods for making your own cream substitutes:

- Whisk silken tofu until smooth for a single cream alternative, loosening it with unsweetened soya milk if necessary.

- To replicate whipped cream, chill a tin of coconut milk, remove the thick top layer and whip it until it holds peaks and has formed a thick cream. Sweeten to taste.

- You can make your own 'cream' with raw nuts – creamy, mild cashews work well. Blitz soaked raw, unsalted nuts in a high-powered blender with a little water until smooth and creamy. Strain through muslin or a clean cloth if desired. Use in dressings, and to make ice cream. (Bear in mind that nut cream isn't whippable.) To make it mimic soured cream, add lemon or lime juice and nutritional yeast to taste.

YOGHURTS

Most vegan yoghurts are made with cashews, almonds, soya beans or coconut milk and can be found on the chilled aisle. Coconut and soya yoghurts are particularly rich and smooth. They are available plain or sweetened and flavoured. Most contain live yoghurt cultures to give them the familiar lactic tang, and added vitamins and calcium. Use in dips, dressings and serve with puddings, fruit or for breakfast, and opt for creamy coconut yoghurt in curries.

Nutritional yeast

Also known as *Saccharomyces cerevisiae* or 'nooch', nutritional yeast has a cheese-like, nutty taste and is a valuable ingredient in the vegan diet. The yeast is grown on molasses (treacle) that has been enriched with minerals and bacteria-grown B_{12}, then dried to deactivate it. It is available in large flakes or a fine powder and adds an umami flavour to savoury foods.

NUTRITIONAL BENEFITS
Rich in protein, minerals and B vitamins.

SERVING SUGGESTIONS
Use the flakes as a substitute for grated Parmesan in pasta dishes and savoury bakes, sprinkle the flakes over popcorn, oven-baked kale chips or roasted vegetables; add a little powder to stocks for soups or rice; coat sliced tofu with powder and soy sauce; add the powder to the sauce for a vegan mac 'n' cheese; add a sprinkle of powder to a slow-cooked lentil stew.

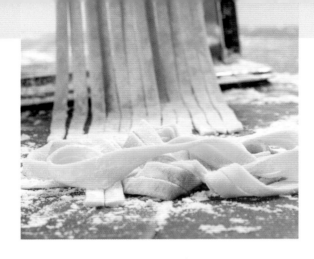

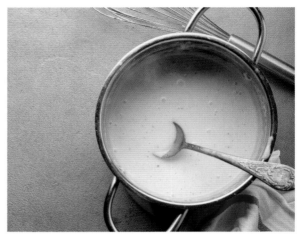

Recipes

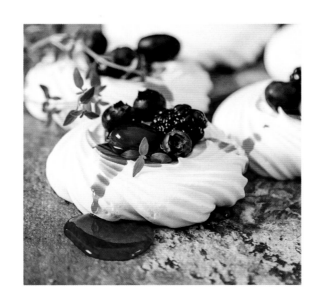

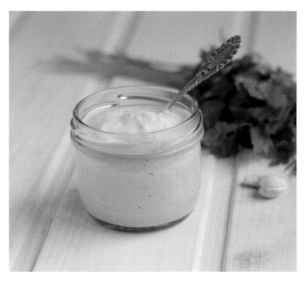

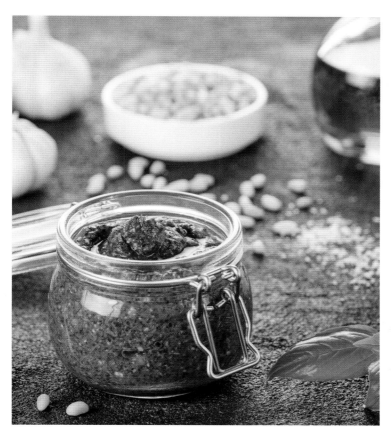

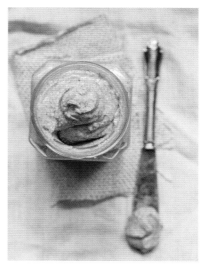

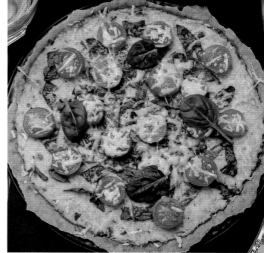

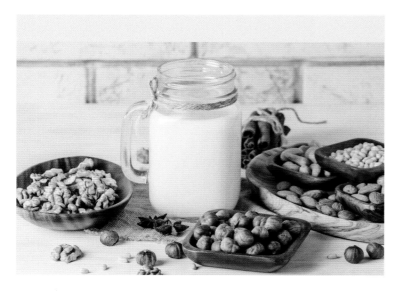

VEGETABLE STOCK

You can use virtually any leafy green vegetables, root vegetables, beans and alliums in a healthy home-made vegetable stock. Use the stock for soups, casseroles, stews, curries and risottos, or savoury sauces and gravy.

MAKES: about 2 litres (3½ pints)

INGREDIENTS:

1 large onion, chopped (with its skin)

3 garlic cloves, chopped (with their skins)

trimmings from up to eight of the following vegetables – leek, celery, celeriac, fennel, carrot, turnip, parsnip, swede, beetroot, potato, sweet potato, butternut squash, courgette, mangetout, broad beans, cabbage, kale, spinach, Swiss chard

a small handful or a few sprigs of two of the following herbs – coriander (leaves and stems), parsley, sage, thyme, rosemary, oregano, fennel, bay leaves

one of the following spices, to taste – sliced fresh ginger root, turmeric root, a star anise, whole cloves, grated nutmeg, a small stick of cinnamon

1 tsp black peppercorns

2 tbsp white wine or cider vinegar

1–2 tsp sea salt

METHOD:

1 Put the vegetables, herbs and spice in a large heavy saucepan. Add the peppercorns, vinegar and 2 litres (3½ pints) cold water. Cover with a lid and set over a high heat.

2 When the water comes to the boil, reduce the heat to a gentle simmer and cook for at least 2–3 hours, stirring occasionally and checking that there's enough liquid. Top up with more water if necessary.

3 When the stock smells really aromatic, remove the pan from the heat. Add sea salt to taste and leave, covered, in a cool place (not the fridge) overnight. The flavour will become more intense as it cools down.

4 The following day, strain the stock through a large sieve. Discard the vegetables and herbs and pour the strained stock into clean glass jars or plastic containers. Cover and keep in the fridge for up to 5 days or in the freezer for up to 2 months.

BÉCHAMEL SAUCE

Being a vegan doesn't mean you have to go without a creamy, savoury white sauce. The method is the same as a classic dairy-based white sauce – all you do is swap the butter for olive oil and use non-dairy milk.

MAKES: 400ml (14fl oz)

INGREDIENTS:

1 tbsp olive oil

30g (1oz) plain flour

400ml (14fl oz) unsweetened nut milk, warmed

a good pinch of freshly grated nutmeg

sea salt and freshly ground black pepper

METHOD:

1 Heat the oil in a saucepan set over a medium heat and stir in the flour with a wooden spoon. Keep stirring until they combine in to a smooth ball.

2 Add a little of the warmed milk and whisk until well combined. Keep adding the milk, a little at a time, whisking between each addition until smooth.

3 When all the milk has been added, increase the heat and keep stirring until the mixture comes to the boil and thickens. Reduce the heat and stir in the nutmeg and some sea salt and black pepper to taste.

NOTE:

To make cheese sauce: make the béchamel sauce following the recipe above. Stir in 1–2 tsp Dijon mustard and 2 tbsp nutritional yeast. For a more intense flavour, you could also add some shredded vegan cheese.

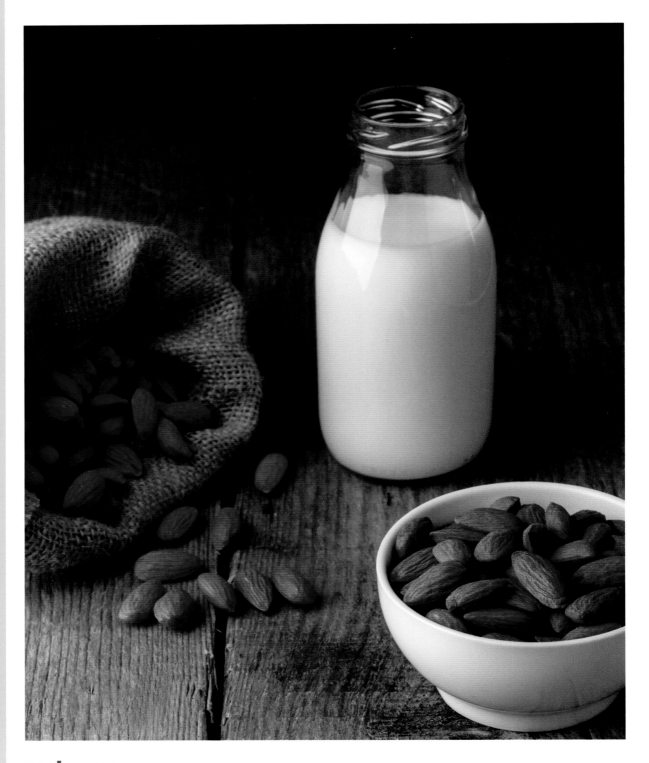

ALMOND MILK

Unsweetened almond milk is low in calories and very nutritious. Although it's lower in protein than cow's milk and soy milk, it has less carbohydrate and contains no saturated fat or sugar, plus it's rich in vitamin E.

MAKES: 600ml (1 pint)

INGREDIENTS:
150g (5oz) raw almonds (skin on)

500ml (17fl oz) filtered water

METHOD:
1 Put the almonds in a bowl and pour over enough cold tap water to cover them. Cover and leave to soak in a cool place for 8–12 hours or overnight– they will get plumper as they absorb the water.

2 The following day, drain the almonds in a colander or sieve, then rinse thoroughly under cold running water. Peel off the skins and discard.

3 Put the almonds in a blender with the filtered water. Cover securely and blitz at high speed for 2–3 minutes until well blended and smooth.

4 Line a strainer with a muslin cloth and place over a measuring jug. Press the almond mixture through the muslin, squeezing it to extract all the liquid.

5 Pour the strained nut milk into sterilized bottles or airtight containers. Seal and store in the fridge for up to 5 days. Shake well before using.

NOTE:
For chocolate milk, blitz the almond milk with 1 tbsp vegan cocoa powder.

RICE MILK

This nutritious and tasty alternative to nut milk is cheaper than store-bought versions, and – as a natural source of carbohydrate – is naturally sweet.

MAKES: 600ml (1 pint)

INGREDIENTS:
115g (4oz) brown rice, cooked

500ml (17fl oz) filtered water

METHOD:
1 Put the cooked rice and water in a blender. Cover securely and blitz at high speed for 2–3 minutes until well blended and smooth.

2 Line a sieve with a clean muslin cloth and place over a measuring jug. Press the rice mixture through the muslin, squeezing it to extract all the liquid.

3 Pour the strained rice milk into sterilized bottles or airtight containers. Seal and store in the fridge for up to 4 days.

NOTE:
You can use white rice instead of brown, but it has less flavour and fewer nutrients.

tip

If you plan to make all your own plant milks, it's worth investing in a reusable nut milk bag, which is designed specifically for the purpose. Many health and whole food stores stock them, or you can buy one online.

NUT BUTTER

By making your own nut butters, you can get the flavour and texture you really like while avoiding palm oil, sugar and other additives that are found in many commercial brands. For the best results, use shelled raw nuts and roast them in the oven.

MAKES: 500g (18oz)

INGREDIENTS:

500g (18oz) shelled raw nuts, such as peanuts, cashews, almonds, macadamia nuts

1 tbsp sunflower, vegetable or groundnut oil

sea salt or Himalayan salt to taste (optional)

1–2 tbsp agave syrup (optional)

METHOD:

1 Preheat the oven to 180°C (160°C fan/350°F/Gas 4).

2 Spread the nuts out on a large baking tray and roast for 10–15 minutes until golden brown and fragrant. Remove from the oven and leave to cool.

3 Blitz the cold nuts in a food processor until coarse and gritty. At this stage, remove 3–4 spoonfuls if you want a crunchy nut butter.

4 With the motor running, add the oil gradually through the feed tube, stopping occasionally and removing the lid to scrape down the sides of the bowl, and continue blitzing until the nuts release their oils and you have a moist, creamy paste. This can take around 10–15 minutes. Stir in the coarsely ground nuts, if you removed them earlier, together with salt and agave to taste (if using).

5 Transfer the nut butter to a sterilized 500g (18oz) glass jar with a screw-top lid, or a Mason jar, and store in the fridge for up to 2 months.

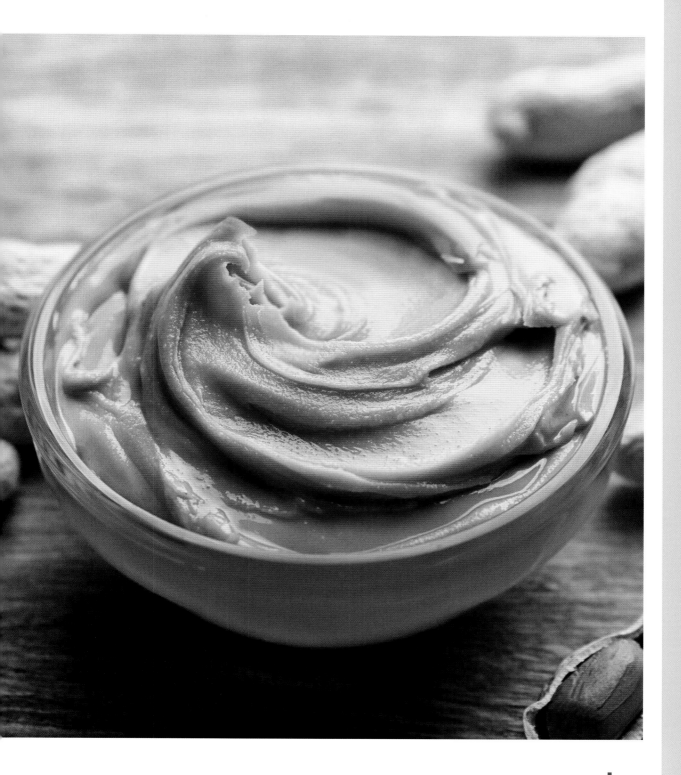

MAYONNAISE

Aquafaba is the Italian word for 'bean water' and you can make a delicious, thick and silky-textured mayonnaise by substituting aquafaba (the liquid from a drained can of chickpeas) for eggs.

MAKES: 250ml (9fl oz)

INGREDIENTS:
50ml (2fl oz) aquafaba (liquid from 400g/14oz can of chickpeas)

1 tbsp Dijon mustard

a generous pinch of salt

200ml (7fl oz) organic groundnut, olive, avocado, sunflower or rapeseed oil

1 tbsp white wine vinegar or lemon juice

METHOD:

1 Put the aquafaba, mustard and salt in a blender or a grease-free mixing bowl. Blend on high or beat with a hand-held electric whisk until frothy.

2 Now, with the blender motor running, start adding the oil slowly in a thin, steady stream (through the feed tube if using a blender). Keep blending until the consistency is thick and creamy. If using a hand-held whisk, pour the oil very slowly and consistently from a jug, beating all the time.

3 When all the oil has been added, pour in the vinegar or lemon juice and beat in briefly. Taste the mayonnaise to check for seasoning, adding more salt, mustard or vinegar/juice if needed.

4 Transfer to a bowl and use immediately, or store in a covered plastic container in the fridge. It will keep for at least 1 week.

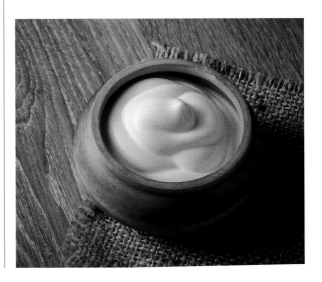

MERINGUE

You only need the drained liquid from one can of chickpeas to make delicious meringues. When you whip chickpea brine it becomes think and fluffy and is a great substitute for beaten egg whites.

INGREDIENTS:

150ml (5fl oz) aquafaba (liquid from 400g/14oz can of chickpeas)

225g (8oz) caster sugar

1½ tsp cream of tartar

fresh berries and grated chocolate, to serve

METHOD:

1 Preheat the oven to 110°C (90°C fan/230°F/Gas ¼). Trace a 23cm (9in) circle on a sheet of baking paper and use to line a baking tray.

2 Pour the aquafaba into a grease-free bowl of an electric mixer (or a deep, grease-free mixing bowl if using a hand-held electric whisk). Start whisking on a slow speed and gradually increase to high speed, for 3–5 minutes until fluffy and soft peaks form.

3 Thoroughly combine the sugar and cream of tartar in a small bowl and then start adding it to the aquafaba, about 2 tablespoons at a time, whisking on a high speed until it has all been incorporated. Keep whisking until the meringue is thick and glossy, with stiff peaks that hold their shape.

4 Drop heaped spoonfuls (about 12) of the meringue mixture onto a lined baking tray and cook in the preheated oven.

5 Bake for 2 hours, until the meringue is crisp and dry on the outside, then turn off the oven, open the door slightly so it's ajar and leave the meringue inside for 30–45 minutes until cool.

6 Serve with fresh berries and grated chocolate.

SHORTCRUST PASTRY

This vegan pastry recipe is so simple: you just throw everything into the food processor and blitz (you can also make it by hand if you don't have a food processor). The olive oil makes the pastry light and easy to handle.

MAKES: 300g (10oz)

INGREDIENTS:

300g (10oz) wholemeal flour, plus extra for dusting

90ml (3fl oz) light olive oil

a pinch of sea salt

METHOD:

1 Put the flour in the food processor bowl and add the olive oil. Blitz until it resembles fine breadcrumbs. Add 60ml (2fl oz) cold water and the salt and pulse briefly until the mixture binds together and you have a soft, not sticky, dough. If you don't have a food processor just put the flour in a large mixing bowl and use your fingertips to rub the oil into the flour and salt before stirring in the water and mixing well.

2 Turn out the pastry onto a lightly floured surface and gently bring it together into a smooth ball. For the best results, handle it lightly and take care not to over-work it.

3 Wrap the dough tightly in clingfilm and leave to rest in the fridge for 30 minutes before using.

tip

This pastry freezes well, so you could make double the quantity and freeze one portion to use at a later date. It will keep in the freezer for up to 3 months. Thaw overnight in the fridge before using.

PESTO

Pesto is much more than just a sauce for tossing pasta with – it also doubles up as a dip or a dressing and can be added to sauces. The nutritional yeast gives the pesto its authentic cheesy flavour and is a great source of minerals and vitamins such as B$_{12}$.

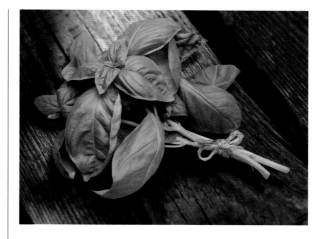

MAKES: about 100g (3½oz)

INGREDIENTS:

50g (2oz) fresh basil

4 tbsp pine nuts

4 garlic cloves, peeled

3 tbsp nutritional yeast

¼ tsp sea salt

juice of ½ lemon

4 tbsp extra-virgin olive oil

METHOD:

1 Pick the stalks off the basil leaves and place the leaves in a blender or food processor with the pine nuts, garlic, nutritional yeast, sea salt and lemon juice. Blitz on high speed until blended to a thick paste.

2 With the motor running, add the olive oil in a thin stream through the feed tube followed by 4 tbsp water, a spoonful at a time, until you have the right consistency – it shouldn't be too thick nor too thin.

3 Use immediately or pour into a sterilized screw-top jar. Cover the pesto with a little olive oil to help keep it fresh, seal and store in the fridge for up to 1 week. The pesto may discolour a little over time, but it will be magically enhanced when you give it a good stir.

VEGAN CREAM CHEESE

This tangy cream cheese is so versatile. Add the flavourings of your choice and you'll have a delicious savoury or sweet cream cheese.

Soaking the cashews gives the cheese a smooth and creamy texture. Don't skip this important step – plan ahead and soak the cashews overnight so they're ready to go the following day.

MAKES: 350g (12oz)

INGREDIENTS:

225g (8oz) raw cashews

120ml (4fl oz) coconut cream

1 tbsp lemon juice

1 tbsp white or cider vinegar

1 tsp sea salt

METHOD:

1 Put the cashews in a heatproof bowl and cover them with boiling water. Leave to soak for at least 2 hours (preferably overnight), then drain well.

2 Put the soaked cashews in a powerful blender with the coconut cream, lemon juice, vinegar and salt and blitz until smooth, thick and creamy. Scrape the mixture down from the sides of the blender bowl occasionally to ensure everything is well blended and you don't end up with any lumps.

3 Taste for seasoning and add more salt, lemon juice or vinegar if desired.

4 Transfer the cream cheese to a bowl, cover and chill in the fridge for a few hours or preferably overnight before using. It will keep in the fridge for up to 1 week (or in the freezer for up to 1 month).

tip

If you are on a low-sodium diet or want to serve this cream cheese with a dessert, you may wish to reduce the amount of salt used.

FRESH PASTA

Most fresh pasta is made with eggs, but you can make delicious eggless pasta yourself at home and you don't need a pasta machine to achieve good results.

MAKES: 400g (14oz) pasta

INGREDIENTS:

300g (10oz) semolina flour, plus extra for dusting

½ tsp salt

150ml (5fl oz) tepid water

2 tbsp olive oil

METHOD:

1 Combine the flour and salt in a large mixing bowl. Make a well in the centre and pour in the tepid water and oil. Mix well with a round-bladed knife to form a smooth dough that leaves the sides of the bowl clean. If it's too dry, add a little more tepid water; if it's too sticky, add some more flour.

2 Turn the dough out onto a lightly floured surface and knead for about 10 minutes until soft and smooth. When kneading, fold the dough inwards towards you with one hand while pushing it away from you with the other. Don't be gentle – you need to pull it and stretch it.

3 Wrap the dough in clingfilm and chill in the fridge for at least 30 minutes to allow it to rest.

4 If you have a pasta machine, roll out the dough according to the instructions. If you are making the pasta by hand, cut the dough into four pieces and sprinkle with flour. Place one piece on a lightly floured surface, dust with flour and roll out by hand, as thinly as you can, into a long rectangle. Try to get the pasta as thin as a piece of paper.

5 Cut the rolled-out dough into long thin strips – about 6mm (¼in) wide – and leave to dry for 10 minutes. You can drape it over the back of a chair if it's very long! If you cook it when it's really soft and freshly rolled, it will be more likely to stick together in the pan.

6 If you wish, you can shape the strips into a loose cylinder and cut through it with a sharp knife to make little round nests of pasta ready for cooking.

7 Cook the pasta in a large pan of boiling salted water for about 3 minutes until al dente (to the 'bite') – it should be just tender but still slightly firm. Drain well and toss with pesto (see page 167) or the sauce of your choice.

NOTE:

This pasta also freezes well. Just follow the instructions for making pasta nests and freeze them on a tray (to help keep their shape) before transferring to a freezer bag (they will keep for up to 2 months). Cook from frozen.

tip

While you are rolling out the pasta, cover the remaining dough with a cloth to keep it soft and stop it drying out.

PIZZA CRUST

You can make a conventional pizza base with flour, water and oil but if you prefer a low-carb alternative try this cauliflower crust.

MAKES: 2 pizza bases (serves 4–6)

INGREDIENTS:

1 large cauliflower (about 675g/1½lb)

2 tbsp finely ground flaxseeds

5 tbsp warm water

115g (4oz) ground almonds, almond flour, or spelt or white flour

a good pinch of salt

1 garlic clove, crushed

1 tbsp olive oil

METHOD:

1 Preheat the oven to 200°C (180°C fan/400°F/Gas 6). Line two large baking sheets with baking paper.

2 Discard the central stalk and leaves from the cauliflower and separate the head into florets. Put them in a food processor and pulse until they have the consistency of crumbs.

3 Transfer to a glass bowl, cover with clingfilm and microwave on high for 3–4 minutes. If you don't have a microwave, steam until tender. Set aside and when it's cool enough to handle, spoon the cauliflower onto a stack of kitchen paper or a clean tea towel and press out the liquid. Alternatively, place in a piece of clean muslin over a bowl and squeeze.

4 Whisk the ground flaxseeds and warm water in a small bowl. Set aside for at least 5 minutes before using. Better still, chill in the fridge for 15 minutes.

5 Mix the cauliflower with the ground almonds or flour, salt and garlic in a large bowl. Add the flaxseed water and olive oil and stir until the mixture forms a dough-like ball. If it's too dry, add more water; if it's too wet, add more ground almonds or flour.

6 Divide the mixture into two portions and shape each one into a round. Place on the lined baking sheets and flatten and stretch them out with your hands to form 1cm (½in) thick circles.

7 Cook in the preheated oven for 15–20 minutes or until cooked through, golden and crisp around the edges.

8 Remove from the oven and turn up the temperature to 230°C (210°C fan/450°F/ Gas 8). Add the topping of your choice, such as home-made tomato sauce, pitted black olives, sautéed mushrooms, roasted peppers and vegan cheese, and bake in the oven for 5–10 minutes before cutting into slices.

tip

Flax 'eggs' are made by whisking freshly ground flax seeds with water to bind the cauliflower mixture.

BIBLIOGRAPHY

1. Darmadi-Blackberry, I., Wahlqvist, M.L., Kouris-Blazos, A., Steen, B., Lukito, W., Horie, Y., Horie, K. 'Legumes: the most important dietary predictor of survival in older people of different ethnicities'. *Asia Pacific Journal of Clinical Nutrition* (2004).

2. Craig, W.J. 'Health effects of vegan diets'. *American Journal of Clinical Nutrition* (2009).

3. Barnard, N., Levin, S., Trapp, C. 'Meat Consumption as a risk factor for Type 2 Diabetes'. *Nutrients* (2014).
Bouvard, V., Loomis, D., Guyton, K.Z., Grosse, Y., El Ghissassi, F., Benbrahim-Tallaa, L., Guha, N., Mattock, H., Straif, K. 'Carcinogenicity of consumption of red and processed meat'. *The Lancet Oncology* (2015).

4. Cancer Council Australia; National Cancer Control Policy. 'Position Statement: Fruit, vegetables and cancer prevention'. (2014).

5. Miura, K., Stamler, J., Brown, I.J., Ueshima, H., Nakagawa, H., Sakurai, M., Chan, Q., Appel, L.J., Okayama, A., Okuda, N., Curb, J.D., Rodriguez, B.L., Robertson, C., Zhao, L., Elliott, P. 'Relationship of dietary monounsaturated fatty acids to blood pressure: the international study of macro/micronutrients and blood pressure'. *Journal of Hypertension* (2013).

6. Sacks, F.M., Lichtenstein, A.H., Wu, J.H.Y., Appel, L.J., Creager, M.A., Kris-Etherton, P.M., Miller, M., Rimm, E.B., Rudel, L.L., Robinson, J.G., Stone, N.J., Van Horn, L.V. 'Dietary Fats and Cardiovascular Disease: A Presidential Advisory from the American Heart Association'. *Circulation* (2017).

7. Ahmed, S.H., Guillem, K., Vandaele, Y. 'Sugar addiction: pushing the drug-sugar analogy to the limit'. *Current Opinion in Clinical Nutrition and Metabolic Care* (2013).

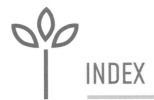

INDEX

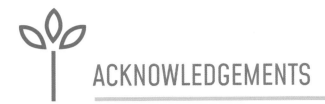

ACKNOWLEDGEMENTS

ABOUT THE AUTHORS

Rose Glover is a vegan nutritional therapist. She runs a consultancy that guides and supports women with varying ailments. She is particularly interested in the link between hormones, digestion, sleep and immune issues and having a plant-based diet. More information on her can be found at www.roseglovernutrition.com.

Laura Nickoll is an editor, food and restaurant writer. She is a member of the Guild of Food Writers, judge for the Great Taste Awards and contributing author to the *Where Chefs Eat* restaurant guides and *The Science of Spice*.

PICTURE CREDITS

ShutterstockPhotoInc. 2–3 Rimma Bondarenko; 4–5 Romariolen; 6–7 Oleksandra Naumenko; 8 Diana Taliun (pea pods); 8 Antonina Vlasova (milks); 8 Fascinadora (jar); 9 Lost Mountain Studio (grains); 9 Yevgeniya Shal (asparagus); 9 Nopparat Promtha (grains in spoons); 9 Nina Firsova (coconut); 9 Eugenia Lucasenco (avocados); 11 Rimma Bondarenko; 19 Eskymaks (tofu); 19 Markus Mainka (chickpeas); 21 nadianb; 26 Jiri Hera; 27 Elena Veselova; 30 Sunny Forest ; 30–1 denio109; 38 zkruger (lentils); 38 Valerii_Dex (mango); 38 nesavinov (spinach); 38 Andy Wasley (tomatoes); 39 Magdalena Kucova (parsley); 39 Diana Taliun (beans); 39 Secha (tomato sauce); 39 HelloRF Zcool (avocados); 41 almaje; 43 QinJin; 44 Foxys Forest Manufacture; 46 Dionisvera (cumin seeds); 46 Medolka (tomatoes); 46 tarapong srichaiyos (garlic); 46 Tatiana Frank (aubergine); 47 mama_mia (sweet potatoes); 47 Maly Designer (spring onion); 47 olepeshkina (kale); 47–8 Svetlana Lukienko (leafy greens); 47 Nedim Bajramovic (turnips); 51 Ivanna Pavliuk; 52 stockcreations (potatoes); 52 Anna Chavdar (vegetables on wooden table); 52–3 Valentina_G (beetroot and carrots); 53 sarsmis (parsnips); 53 Sabino Parente (celeriac); 53 istentiana (vegetables in wooden box); 56–7 STUDIO GRAND WEB; 60 BEAUTY STUDIO; 60–1 Natasha Breen; 64–5 Fedorovacz; 68 Ferumov (wild garlic); 68 NUM LPPHOTO (shallots); 68 Nicole Agee (vegetables in box); 73 Tim UR (cauliflower); 73 images72 (savoy cabbage); 73 Alexander Prokopenko (red cabbage); 76–7 Azdora; 82 Africa Studio (asparagus); 82 abamjiwa al-hadi (corn); 82 KarepaStock (artichokes); 82–3 5 second Studio (fennel); 83 frank60 (okra); 83 ArtCookStudio (celery); 85 Avdeyukphoto; 88 Magdanatka; 89 JL-Pfeifer (mangetout); 89 AnaMarques (runner beans); 89 PosiNote (green beans); 89 Sea Wave (green peas); 91 Fernando Sanchez Cortes (sea lettuce); 91 Amarita (dried seaweed); 93 marco mayer; 96 Amawasri Pakdara; 98 inewsfoto; 100–1 margouillat photo; 105 kostrez (red and green lentils); 105 bitt24 (lentils in wooden bowl); 107 Svetlana Lukienko; 108 Krasula; 110 nabianb; 111 Valentyn Volkov; 117 SMarina (pumpkin seeds); 117 BarthFotografie (sesame seeds); 121 Africa Studio; 123 Evgeny Karandaev; 126 Africa Studio (flour); 126 Greentellect Studio (barley); 126 New Africa (flour); 127 StockImageFactory.com (semolina); 127 everydayplus (quinoa); 127 Vezzani Photography (popcorn); 129 Vladislav Noseek (oats); 130 GreenTree (grains); 131 Brent Hofacker; 132 Pavlo Lys; 136 bigacis; 138–9 Dionisvera; 142–3 fotoknips; 145 grafvision; 147 HandmadePictures; 148 zygonema; 150 Julia Sudnitskaya; 156 fototip (pasta); 156 Olha Afanasieva (béchamel sauce); 156 Gaus Alex (meringue); 156 Svetlana Zelentsova (mayonnaise); 157 Fascinadora (pesto); 157 Magdalena Paluchowska (butter); 157 Goskova Tatiana (milk); 157 Nataliya Arzamasova (pizza); 160 Lana_M; 163 Africa Studio; 164 Bekshon; 167 Billion Photos.

EDDISON BOOKS LIMITED
Managing Director Lisa Dyer
Commissioning Editor Victoria Marshallsay
Managing Editor Nicolette Kaponis
Copy Editor Laura Nickoll
Proofreader Claire Rogers
Indexer Angie Hipkin
Designer Louise Evans
Production Gary Hayes